# Health Care and the Autism Spectrum

WITHDRAWN

# Health Care and the Autism Spectrum

A Guide for Health Professionals, Parents and Carers

*Alison Morton-Cooper*

Jessica Kingsley Publishers
London and Philadelphia

First published in the United Kingdom in 2004
by Jessica Kingsley Publishers
116 Pentonville Road
London N1 9JB, UK
and
400 Market Street, Suite 400
Philadelphia, PA 19106, USA

*www.jkp.com*

Copyright © Jessica Kingsley Publishers 2004

Second impression 2005

**Library of Congress Cataloging in Publication Data**

Morton-Cooper, Alison.
  Health care and the autism spectrum / Alison Morton-Cooper.— 1st
American pbk. ed.
    p. cm.
Includes bibliographical references and index.
  ISBN 1-85302-963-7 (pbk.)
  1. Autism. 2. Medical care. I. Title.
  RC553.A88M68 2004
  616.85'882—dc22

                                                              2003026858

**British Library Cataloguing in Publication Data**
A CIP catalogue record for this book is available from the British Library

ISBN-13: 978 1 85302 963 9
ISBN-10: 1 85302 963 7

Printed and Bound in Great Britain by
Athenaeum Press, Gateshead, Tyne and Wear

WITHDRAWN

# Contents

# Acknowledgements

Many people have contributed to this book by sharing personal experiences and 'stories' together with the wisdom and insight they have acquired from being at the front line of health care practice and the care of their loved ones.

I would first of all like to acknowledge the inspiration, expertise and unconditional support offered by a strong parents' support group, and in particular the help of Karen Priestley, Laura Dykes and all friends who regularly attend our meetings. Robert Mackay and colleagues from the National Autistic Society (Scotland) have always been a ready source of support, information and guidance for which I'm extremely grateful.

Turning an idea or personal conviction into a reality is always a challenge for authors who embark on the 'long and winding road' to publication. In this case the road had more twists and turns in it than was ever expected, largely because of a dearth of available peer-reviewed literature and the frustration felt when a need is recognised and there seem to be few 'signposts' to suggest a clear way to meet it. Changes in my own personal circumstances as this book came to fruition also prompted a major review of the important things in life, not least about how vital it is to nurture and maintain support and communication networks when life throws up surprises and challenges for which we perhaps feel unprepared.

Many health and social care professionals have made available their time and enthusiasm to listen and to share their own insights and resources.

I would like to thank Allison Richardson (former specialist health visitor), Jill McKean (occupational therapist and 'whiz' on sensory integration problems), Pam Edgar, Margaret Brown and colleagues from the

Children with Disabilities team from Dumfries & Galloway Council's social work department, and Claudine Brindle of the Princess Royal Trust for Carers, Dumfries, all of whom have contributed in their own special ways, largely by providing tactical support and encouragement when it was needed most. Their professionalism, empathy and kindness continue to be much appreciated.

I'm also grateful for the support of colleagues in the library and information services, especially Anne Glencross, recently retired administrator of the Post-Graduate Medical Centre and Library at Dumfries & Galloway Royal Infirmary (NHS Dumfries and Galloway), and former colleagues at the University of Glasgow's Crichton Campus in Dumfries.

Surviving and thriving has also depended on the very high standard of care and attention given to my family by local family doctors, Lois Sproat, Jim Duck and all colleagues at the Castle Douglas Medical Group. A rural practice it may be, but at the cutting edge of best practice as far as my family is concerned. The expertise of specialist physiotherapist Janet Leith and colleagues of 'Revive Scotland' in Glasgow has also kept me on the move when my body might have felt like doing otherwise!

I would also like to thank Dr Margaret Bamford, my long-time mentor and friend, for all her love and support. My mother, Bessie Morton, has also 'been there' whenever the need has arisen, despite difficulties with her own health and those within the extended family. My husband Barrie and son Alastair and all supporters within the family (they know who they are!) know how much their love and encouragement has meant to me.

I am enormously grateful to Jessica Kingsley and all colleagues at JKP for their patience, understanding and expertise. Breaking new ground is never easy and having the courage to share my conviction will I hope be repaid when the special health care needs of people with autism begin to be seriously acknowledged in health care practice.

Finally I would like to dedicate this book to the memory of my friend and former nursing tutor/co-author, Professor Anne Palmer, who sadly died in the spring of 2003, just as her extraordinary gifts as a teacher were coming into their fullest flower.

Her guiding principle was always to see the best in people and to enable them to develop their talents in ways that would change the world for the better. Health care has been the richer for her contribution and energy and I know she will be with me in spirit for this my latest 'adventure'.

*Alison Morton-Cooper,*
*Castle Douglas, 2003*

# Introduction

The volume and range of medical services available in the UK National Health Service and in the private sector can be daunting for most people. For a person with a pervasive developmental and communication difficulty, gaining access to medical help and obtaining the right health care often depends on the support and advice available to them in their particular home setting. In the case of people with autism this can range from a traditional family home to residential accommodation (designated special schools or care homes), or to living with foster families or in supported accommodation in the community. Some may live alone, while others will be in long-term relationships and may have children or be step-parents. Those who have not had their communication difficulties properly recognised or diagnosed may be living and sleeping rough, or may have found their way into custodial care and been deprived of their liberty because of their inability to communicate their intentions appropriately.

Psychologist Rita Jordan warns that while people with obvious learning disabilities may have received some level of understanding of their difficulties, the more able person with autism who seems (superficially) to be able to communicate well may have devised strategies that disguise their real problems so that their residual difficulties are misunderstood. As she explains, they may attract more potentially harmful labels, such as being lazy, rude or even aggressive. 'Bewildered by the hostility and lack of support they receive, they may lose their carefully constructed coping behaviours and could end up excluded from the service' (Jordan 1999, p.115). She writes that undiagnosed pupils with autism often end in schools for pupils with emotional and behavioural difficulties and then may not have access to required special provision for autism. 'Undiagnosed adults may end up on the streets or even in prison because their behaviour is misunderstood and they are vulnerable to manipulation by others,' she warns (p.115).

The quality and kind of health care people with an autism spectrum condition receive will depend not only on the interpretation of their needs by others close to them, but also on how autism-aware frontline health care workers are and how sympathetic and attuned they may be to modifying their usual practice to accommodate communication and sensory problems.

Few primary care trusts, hospitals, clinics or health facilities have specific policies or guidelines pertaining to the care of people with autism, although most (sadly of necessity) have a policy for managing violent or aggressive patients. The basic tenets of good interpersonal communication – polite and considerate behaviour (Bornat 1999) – are not always within the remit of people with autism. Struggling to understand and to make oneself understood takes up enormous amounts of physical and emotional energy. A lack of social awareness and ability to relate to others lies at the core of autism as a disability. Busy health professionals don't usually have time to dissect language and social interaction and have to work within widely accepted norms and values. Toleration of difference does not usually extend to accepting aggression or physical/verbal abuse unless a clear physiological explanation attends an emotional outburst (such as head injury or stroke).

Edgar Schneider, who has been diagnosed with high functioning autism and attention deficit disorder, eloquently expresses his own difficulties in relating to others:

> First, as far as being able to connect with other live human beings, male or female, I am an emotional idiot [sic]. (That last phrase is mine; the phrase commonly used in psychology is emotional deficit.) It seems that, just as some people have an important physical component missing (eyes, limbs, etc.), I have an important component of the human psyche missing: the ability to connect emotionally with other human beings. This, however, may be somewhat simplistic. We are not automata, totally devoid of all feeling. What we lack are the emotions that enable people to 'connect' with the emotions of other people. I do find myself as having experienced what I call the 'survival' emotions: fear and anger. The

fact that autism takes away the social, connective emotions, but leaves the survival emotions, sometimes rendering one asocial, could be considered as one of Mother Nature's sick jokes. (Schneider 1999, p.25)[1]

The autism community has a tremendous affection for the character Data in the television sci-fi series Star Trek simply because as an android, ostensibly devoid of human emotion and motivation, his skills of rational decision making and lack of emotional hinterland are great assets when taking on interplanetary conflicts. His attempts at understanding human relationships are poignant and touching to watch for those of us who live with people who have autism, because his character demonstrates quite graphically how very difficult it is to gain access to human emotions if they have been denied by neurological (or in his case mechanical!) impairment. To people with autism, Data is something of a folk hero because he verbalises many of the internal conflicts they feel in trying to make sense of the world. An important caveat needs to be stressed here, however. It isn't a lack of feeling that is the problem in autism, but rather a difficulty in expressing feelings appropriately and in context.

Clearly, hospital and health trust policies are unlikely to have taken in the subtle nuances of Data's struggle with the world. Frontline workers in health care – that is, the receptionists, clerks, hospital porters, ambulance drivers, nursing and medical staff and professionals allied to medicine – will all have their own idea of what it means to have an autism perspective on the world. To begin to make sense of it and to understand how practice needs to be modified accordingly needs further study and consideration. I hope at least that some of the suggestions and strategies discussed in this book will provide a basic framework for action.

Chapter 1 gives an overview of autism and associated problems with health care. The remaining chapters are arranged according to different types of contact with health and social care services. Chapter 2 deals with the issue of health care and autism from the perspective of primary care

---

1    Excerpt from *Discovering My Autism: Apologia Pro Vita Sua (with Apologies to Cardinal Newman)* (1999) by Edgar Schneider is reprinted by permission of Jessica Kingsley Publishers, London. © 1999 Edgar Schneider.

consultation. Chapters 3–5 will be more concerned with aspects of care in acute care settings, such as hospitals and specialist services. Finally, Chapter 6 looks at some issues of social and community support. Each area considered is complex once you begin to analyse the issues and potential challenges, so what I have attempted to do is to crystallise the key questions and practical aspects from my own reading of the literature available, together with insights picked up from my professional and personal experience and those shared with me by colleagues, friends and families affected by the autism spectrum. It is my hope that this will stimulate further interest in the subject amongst health and social care professionals so that the literature and related guidelines will be added to over time.

# 1 How This Book Can Help

This book is for health professionals who need to know more about how the nursing, medical and health care needs of a person with an autism spectrum disorder may be met. The spectrum of autism comprises impairments in social interaction, communication and imagination, which vary in severity in different individuals. I shall refer to this range of conditions generally as 'autism' throughout this book.

## About autism

### The basics

Although a great deal of research and study of autism and its causes, epidemiology and diagnostic criteria has been carried out since the condition was first described by Leo Kanner and Hans Asperger in the 1940s, even now, as the recognition and accuracy of diagnosis is steadily improving, many people still go undiagnosed and misunderstood in society. The UK National Autistic Society estimates a prevalence rate of 91 per 10,000 of the population for an autism spectrum condition. With an average GP's list of 2000 people, every family doctor is therefore likely to have up to 18 people with autism on their list (National Autistic Society 1999).

Whether or not there is a formal diagnosis depends very much on local awareness and availability of diagnostic services. Until recently autism received little attention within the curricula of medical and nursing schools, so knowledge of the subject among health professionals is often patchy at best. Accurate and up-to-date knowledge of autism and related disorders can't be taken for granted, as a recent study of general practitioners in Glasgow has found (Brogan 2001).

Changes in public attitudes to disability, and government policies that stress social inclusion and care in the community, make it much more likely nowadays that children and young people are cared for within the family home or by foster carers, although some are cared for in specialist residential schools. Most recently diagnosed children (regardless of level of disability) are likely to be educated in mainstream schooling in the UK, unless other complex physical and learning disabilities (or exceptional family circumstances) make specialist schooling essential. It is not unusual for siblings or at least one parent to have some autistic 'features' (known as the 'broad autism phenotype': for an explanation see Howlin 1998). This can obviously complicate matters considerably. Some children with quite profound difficulties are home-educated with a variable level of support from their local education authority.

On the basis of the first generation of people to be formally diagnosed (now in their 50s), predictions as to a long-term future are difficult to generalise. Depending on their level of coping and intellectual abilities, adults with autism may live independently or in accommodation supported by social services in the community. Those at the more able end of the spectrum – sometimes described as having 'high functioning autism' or Asperger's syndrome (AS) – may have long-term relationships, go to work and raise families of their own. Part of why autism is described as a 'spectrum' disorder is because of the huge variations and sheer range of disabilities and capabilities it can represent. People with high functioning autism, for example, have had notable successes in academia, especially in the sciences and engineering and the creative arts where the obsessive interests and strict adherence to routines typical of autistic behaviour are put to positive use (see Jarrold and Routh 1998).

Unless you have a clear understanding of the fundamental deficits of autism, however, you may understandably be deeply puzzled by a condition that affects people so very differently. It should also be borne in mind that although we are used to hearing of the condition in relation to children, as a disorder becoming obvious in later life and in old age, autism is thought to go seriously unrecognised and under-researched.

As anyone who has worked in accident and emergency rooms will know, staff are quite often confronted by distressed and aggressive patients who demonstrate challenging behaviours and find it hard to communicate their needs effectively. It stands to reason that at least some of these will be patients with autism, diagnosed or otherwise. Common sense also suggests that a proportion of the elderly mentally ill in the general population are also likely to be people with undiagnosed autism who have battled through life without the appropriate understanding and support and who remain psychologically, emotionally and perhaps physically damaged as a result.

## Associated medical and dietary problems

Remember that autism is not a psychological problem but a neurological one. People on the autism spectrum may have contributing factors that make care decisions more complicated. Sleep disorders and hyperactivity or, conversely, extreme slowness of movement to the point of catatonia can have implications for care and treatment of medical problems.

Epilepsy is more common than in the general population, and seizures may become apparent at the time of puberty, if not before. It is estimated that the rate of epilepsy in autism is around 30–50 per cent by adult life. In an excellent chapter on the health care of adults with autism, Hugh Morgan advises that because of communication difficulties, certain types of seizures may be under-reported, in particular complex partial seizures or childhood absence seizures such as petit-mal (Morgan 1996). Similarly, episodes of 'clicking out' or staring are often commented on by teachers or carers, whereby the person seems to be temporarily 'absent' and unresponsive to the usual prompts. For advice on catatonia and autism see research and comments by Wing and Shah (2000).

Research to date has also suggested that there may be a link between 'symptoms' of autism and abnormal human gut microflora (Bingham 2003), and many parents and affected individuals report dietary problems or food intolerance. This should also be borne in mind during any consultation as it may not only impact on care management and general nutritional status, but on concerns regarding the ability to take medicines or comply with a treatment regime. Specific background information on the science behind these issues is available online from the Food Microbial Sciences Unit at the University of Reading, UK, and from the University of Sunderland's Autism Research Unit's websites.

## Learning difficulties

Reviews of the biology of autism conclude that evidence for an organic cause is overwhelming and it is estimated that up to 75 per cent of all people with autism may present with general learning difficulties, that is with an IQ below 70 (see Jordan 1999).

The degree of learning disability will clearly have an impact on ability to co-operate in the health consultation and future care, although Jordan makes the useful observation that the autism itself is not responsible for producing the intellectual impairment. People with autism can have severe autism and yet have normal or even advanced levels of intellectual functioning.

Where autism and severe learning difficulties do exist alongside one another, it does not necessarily mean that the autism itself will be equally severe (Jordan 2001). This is an important distinction because it implies that children with normal intelligence have a better chance of overcoming some of the problems associated with autism. They may be able to develop skills and strategies that the child with a more complex learning disability would find impossible. (The downside of this in the longer term is that the autism can then be masked or disguised, until the time comes when a stressor is overpowering and typical features of autism are brought to the surface.)

Ascertaining your patient's general level of intellectual functioning is therefore very important when looking not only to help them regarding health advice, but also to estimate how well different communication strategies can be employed to aid mutual understanding.

## Sensory issues

It seems that our interpretation of sensation is individual, and as a result our reactions can be just as individual, even when we experience the same sensory input or information. It is vital that we recognise the links that exist between sensory input and the behaviours that result, particularly as the patient with autism may have very idiosyncratic responses we haven't come across before.

Smith Myles and her co-authors have written a very useful book on Asperger's syndrome and sensory issues that helpfully describes sensory processing and explains the ways in which it affects behaviour directly (Smith Myles *et al.* 2000). They remind us that each sensory input has the potential to evoke a reaction that then results in a behavioural response, even though the response may be to ignore that particular stimulus in favour of another. Hence, when we sense the rain we know to run for cover or put up an umbrella. When we feel too cold we begin to shiver (as a physiological reaction) and then look for ways to warm ourselves up. If we see a large object hurtling towards us our senses help us to realise that it is time to move quickly out of the way. Our inbuilt sensors warn us of impending problems (pain being a good example) and help us to take restorative or avoiding action.

Effective modulation allows us to balance out our responses so that our behaviour matches the requirements of our particular presenting situation. The body's ability to respond is further modified by our motor planning skills, so that we soon learn to move appropriately and smoothly in response to a particular stimulus. People with autism (and particularly with AS) can have problems with motor planning skills (known as 'motor dyspraxia') so that the necessary actions may be slow or ineffective. The neurological threshold for sensory processing is likely to be idiosyncratic in a person with autism, given the biological basis of brain pathology. Hence a low threshold (i.e. hypersensitivity and over-reaction) may occur for some sensory inputs, while a high threshold (hyposensitivity/under-reaction) may be seen in response to others. These can affect different senses differently, so that a person who is very sensitive to auditory stimuli can, conversely, be under-reactive to other stimuli that would be painful to others. While some stimuli may be filtered out, others may predominate and cause fear and a 'fright, flight or fight' response.

Each individual will have their own particular sensitivities and this can appear contradictory. A child or adult may find bright or twinkling lights a source of fascination and comfort while at the same time finding the bright 'strip' lighting of a modern building quite unbearable. A person with autism may have difficulty in filtering or selecting out a particular stimulus for attention, and focus on something that ordinary people would barely notice. (As an example, I once met a distinguished academic whose major interest in life was the refraction of light. It made him a great physicist but didn't do much for his social skills. I was told he would often end a conversation abruptly if he noticed the light fall in an interesting way behind the person talking to him.)

The inability to process sensory information appropriately can lead to dangerous situations. The person unable to tell the difference between a far-away truck and one coming directly towards him is clearly at a disadvantage. Even if they were able to tell the difference, slower processing may mean they would be unable to take avoiding action in time (which the truck driver may have taken for granted). People with autism may become so interested in the shininess and wetness of a puddle that they fail to sense the dangers of nearby traffic.

All of our nervous systems react to stimuli in their own idiosyncratic way, although most of us can probably rely on them to warn us of the greatest potential dangers. The person with autism who has a poor ability to integrate the senses in this way can often appear eccentric, but they are also obviously made more vulnerable. To give you some examples, if you are cold you might close the draughty window or door, put on a sweater, heat up some warming soup or turn up the central heating. The person with autism might do none of these things – he or she may not register the cold or may not have the planning skills to think through an appropriate course of action.

If it is getting dark outside you will probably switch on the lights and close the curtains for privacy. The person with autism may not notice and may carry on doing whatever they were doing until it becomes impossible or until someone else prompts them to take action. Certain foods or fabrics may be avoided because they cause unpleasant sensory reactions. Certain noises may be selected over others or may become unbearable (hypersensitivity to the sound of dogs barking, the noise of vacuum cleaners and to other ordinary household noises is a common problem).

Some people will have a high threshold for some things and a low threshold for others.

The actual processes involved (i.e. registering awareness of a particular sensory input, orientating oneself to its source, interpreting that input, organising a reaction and then executing a response and adapting to it) may be interrupted at any stage so that responses then reflect the sensory integration problem currently being experienced (for an accessible account, see Smith Myles *et al.* 2000). This would tend to support some of the arguments made for autism that it is in essence a disorder of body sense and moving as much as one of cognition and self–other awareness and communication (Donellan and Leary 1995).

Ineffective sensory processing therefore has broad and deep implications for the ability of the person affected to:

- protect him or herself from danger or abuse

- engage in self-care activities such as personal hygiene, dressing appropriately for the weather or social situation, cooking, eating, going to the toilet, and many of the other activities of daily living

- understand and respond appropriately to some of the more physical health care interventions

- manage illness and health care activities

- express sexuality appropriately

- sensitively interact appropriately with peers and others.

It is also important to bear in mind the possibility of additional sensory impairment as this, too, needs to be taken into account. An excellent clinical/educational project in the south of England developed a policy and protocol for the care of patients with sensory impairments with a view to promoting equal opportunities and access for such patients to services, including participating in care and gaining information that would help them to make informed choices about treatments (Soltysiak and O'Shea 2003). 'Sensory impairment' was however limited to visual, auditory and speech impairments, and it would be good to see such protocols extended to include patients with the sensory and communication problems associated with autism. Clearly if your patient has additional sensory impairments, strategies will again have to be modified to compensate for these.

One reported condition that some people with Asperger's syndrome have written about is that of 'synaesthesia', a rare condition (not apparently exclusive to AS) where a person experiences a sensation in one sensory system but then experiences it as another – a phenomenon sometimes described as 'coloured hearing'. Sounds can be accompanied by 'vague sensations of colour, shape, texture, movement, scent or flavour' (Attwood 1998, p.138). The implications of this for the care of patients are hard to plan for, but perhaps an awareness that it can happen is a good beginning.

## Health care problems and autism

The world of clinics, hospitals, doctors' offices, dental surgeries and operating theatres is bewildering and worrying for most people who find themselves ill and in need of treatment. It shouldn't be surprising then that people with autism who find it hard to understand and interpret the ordinary social rules and demands of everyday life can find health care institutions and the expectations of professionals working in them extremely frightening and confusing.

Autism in all its forms is a complex, lifelong neurodevelopmental disorder that can profoundly affect a person's ability to communicate with, and understand the behaviours of, those around them. People with autism find it difficult to communicate their thoughts, feelings and physical sensations in ways that are easy for others to understand; this can render them very vulnerable when illness strikes, or when normal physical development demands attention. People with autism get ill and are prey to the same physical or psychological problems as everyone else. But their ability to respond to their physical needs may be seriously impaired or complicated by coexisting medical conditions related to their neurological dysfunction (such as epilepsy, catatonia, anxiety and depression), by any accompanying learning disability, and by a range of sensory problems that may lower or, conversely, significantly increase their pain threshold and sensitivity to pain signals. The latter can lead to under- or over-reporting of illness and to an increase in anxiety in vulnerable individuals and a subsequent challenge to their coping abilities. Fear, anxiety and distress when you have little or no real grasp of what is happening to you and your body is a very understandable reaction, which can result in defensive behaviours that may alarm health professionals and onlookers trying to deal with a health situation at a critical time (for example, rocking, shouting or 'ranting' against perceived injustices which are usually the result of misinterpretation or disorientation).

Concerns expressed by carers, parents and affected individuals point to a lack of knowledge and insight from health workers about the ways in which autism can affect a person's responses to medical treatment and health care. Parents and carers who have tried to explain and offer strategies to health professionals have sometimes been dismissed for 'fussing' unnecessarily or have been accused of being over-protective. It is only when damage is unwittingly done and the consequences of unintended harm become apparent that health professionals are made more aware of and sensitive to the special impairments of autism.

Problems of literal interpretation of language and misinterpretation of touch and other expressive gestures can lead to tricky altercations between practitioners and patients – as some have found to their cost. For the person affected by autism, even a typical family doctor consultation or visit to the practice nurse can be a traumatic and anxiety-provoking experience with unintended outcomes for those involved.

The risks involved are very real. First there is the risk that the patient may be misunderstood or have their needs misinterpreted. Then there is the risk of misdiagnosis resulting from poor-quality communication. One young man I have heard about spends most of his time on a garden swing (up to seven hours a day), hence he often complains of pains in his bottom and stiffness in his neck and elbows. The type of localised redness, tenderness and injury he demonstrates could be misinterpreted without access to information about his daily pastimes. This demonstrates the importance of knowing as much as you can about the background circumstances of your patient.

Many young people with high functioning autism spend a lot of time with personal computers and show signs of repetitive strain injury. Associated eye strain and headaches are also not unusual. Practical advice to limit this time and find alternative activities will usually be hard to follow through, but at least you can be aware of where problems are likely to come from and manage them accordingly. Picking at wounds, scratching and biting (self and others) can be a problem, and digging in dirt or smearing faeces is quite common among more severely affected children. Antibiotics, tetanus immunisation and close supervision may be needed to help them avoid contracting serious infections.

It is not uncommon for children with autism educated in mainstream schools to miss out on vaccinations because of a previous history of adverse reactions or allergies (school health staff may refer them back to their GP), and for parents to avoid vaccinations for fear of worsening any existing neurological problems. Sensitive enquiry and clear factual information should be offered to encourage parents and their offspring to protect themselves against potential problems.

Because of difficulties with planning and organisation, weak interpersonal communication and a lack of awareness or knowledge of risks to the self and others, the chances of compliance with professional advice may be greatly reduced. This can lead to real difficulties with regard to consent to treatment, ability to follow instructions properly or compliance with a medications regime.

Many people with autism have sensory sensitivities, so that even basic health-needs assessment is an issue. In a person who is exquisitely sensitive to touch, how do you go about taking a blood pressure reading, dressing a wound or conducting a physical examination? What about exposure to anaesthetics, surgery, administering oxygen or intravenous fluids?

Those severely affected by autism may have no concept of health or health professionals and may react to any physical approach from a stranger with suspicion and fear or by turning to comforting rituals such as rocking or flapping their hands. The usual explanations and reassurance offered to patients may not suffice. Even in the most able people with autism, serious communication deficits may remain, though they may be well hidden behind the characteristic stilted, pedantic and over-complex language of the more intellectually able person with autism.

Many health professionals ask why such problems relating to autism are only now being brought to their attention. This may partly be due to raised awareness of autism from media scares over possible damage to young children from multiple vaccines and partly because of better diagnosis and extensive research into autism in recent years.

The very high-profile publicity given to the more severe forms of autism (known as Kanner's autism) has contributed to most people's image of the mute and severely withdrawn child, lost in their own world and usually exhibiting severe behavioural problems, such as banging their head on the wall or screaming uncontrollably. Those most profoundly affected may need care and support in their activities of daily living for the whole of their lives. In the past such people were given up to the care of large-scale mental handicap hospitals, often without an accurate diagnosis of their difficulties. Contact with the outside world was minimal. Any obvious health care problems were usually the responsibility of hospital staff. Expectations were low and the public at large had little experience of what it meant to live or cope with the condition (for a clear and sensitive explanation of autism's history and evolution, see Wing 2001).

The image of the mute withdrawn child is a very powerful one and attracts widespread public attention and sympathy. Whilst this image is true of some people, it does significantly underplay the more outwardly subtle but nevertheless challenging difficulties faced by people whose autism is expressed differently. Autism is often described as an invisible disability, simply because a lot of the time you can't see obvious outward physical signs. Health professionals need to know what to look for and how to avoid the common pitfalls. Once you are experienced and familiar with autism in all its myriad forms, it does become easier to spot the tell-tale signs, and continuing education and awareness campaigns both for health care practitioners and the general public are beginning to have an impact locally, nationally and internationally.

Health screening and surveillance is another area that could usefully be explored in relation to autism. Preventive health measures such as eye care, nutrition, lifestyle advice, accident prevention and home safety, dentistry and podiatry issues all have the potential to be adversely affected by autism (or ignored) if no one is available to take an interest in these matters for a person who may not be aware of his or her needs.

Sexuality is another area requiring further research, since much of the available advice is geared towards people with a learning disability rather than autism itself. Some aspects of sexuality around relationships and behaviour may have been considered (see Gray, Ruble and Dalrymple 2000; Henault 2003), and perhaps also contraception and safe sex advice. But few people seem to have thought about the kinds of support necessary to help a woman with autism who is pregnant and how she might manage pregnancy and childbirth, the acquisition of parenting skills or obtaining sexual health advice and screening for gynaecological conditions and cancers. Prospective fathers with autism also need to be considered. What about the partner with autism thinking about a long-term commitment, marriage or starting a family? Genetic counselling may be needed too. And the issue of homosexuality and autism is also rarely considered or talked about.

First and foremost it should be recognised that children with autism go on to become adults and sometimes parents with autism. Autism is a lifelong condition characterised by an abnormality of brain function leading to difficulties in communicating with and understanding the intentions of others. It can affect more than one member of a family, even though this may not be recognised or accepted within the family unit. Autism has no known single cause and no known cure.

As individuals with autism struggle to understand and conform to society's expectations of them, the stressors that become apparent in their behavioural responses can lead to real difficulties in coping with health care problems and the health care system.

## Psychological health issues

Although I will be focusing on hospital admission for physical health reasons in this book, it is well recognised that people with autism spectrum conditions can have their problems compounded by psychiatric illness. Autism expert Lorna Wing advises that psychiatric illnesses can emerge in adolescence or adult life, with depression occurring most often, and this tends to be associated with the development of some insight and recognition of being different from peers (Wing 2001). Tony Attwood addressed this issue movingly and sensitively in his best-selling book on Asperger's syndrome (Attwood 1998), and Christopher Gillberg discusses the subject in detail in his guide to AS (Gillberg 2002).

Distinguishing different psychiatric disorders from some of the characteristics of autism must be extremely hard to do, given the pervasiveness of a developmental disorder, but specialist knowledge and understanding is improving. Some people diagnosed as having personality disorders or schizophrenia when they were young may now have their diagnosis reviewed and revised if they meet with the criteria for autism, so that the diagnostic rate for adults is likely to continue increasing for some time.

Emotional support for all people with autism begins with trying to gain an understanding of what the world is like from their perspective (even though no two people will express their communication problems in the same way). By being as tolerant as possible and setting manageable boundaries to their unusual behaviour it is possible to reduce the levels of stress and anxiety they feel with subsequent improvements in their behaviour.

One caveat to this that I would add (from a mother's perspective) is that this can also be something of a 'catch 22'. Where this kind of approach has succeeded and outward signs have become less noticeable, 'outsiders' can imagine that the difficulties have lessened and that the person has somehow 'grown out' of their autism. Further understanding and adjustments may not be made and so the pressures and stresses of 'trying to be normal' re-emerge, placing the child, young person or adult under yet more strain, with the risk of regression into withdrawal and the development of depression and anxiety disorders. The risk of suicide also increases, particularly where severe emotional problems are not recognised in time.

Professionals and the public need to understand that autism is lifelong even where it outwardly appears to be 'mild'. Support services and understanding need to be built around this. Remember also that not everyone with a diagnosis of high functioning autism or AS will wish to disclose this to health professionals (or even to acknowledge and accept the diagnosis) and so may attempt to disguise their difficulties. Some families, too, may not wish to acknowledge the diagnosis and where they do, they may experience feelings of guilt or depression, particularly if they have identified autism elsewhere in the family. Most of the families and individuals I have come into contact with have eventually welcomed a formal diagnosis and the explanations and understanding it brings, even though appropriate services and support may not be easy to obtain.

## Developing autism-friendly practice in health care

Acquiring a reliable evidence base for autism-related practice in health care is a massive undertaking that will take many years to develop. Despite the burgeoning literature on autism diagnosis and behavioural management in recent years there remains an alarming lack of literature and evidence on the ways in which people with autism cope with physical illness.

This book is a tentative first attempt to bring health and social care professionals' attention to the problems autism presents in everyday clinical practice. Inevitably it raises many more questions than it has answers to (a sign of a literature waiting to be born, maybe?) and is intended to help in three ways:

- by providing a short, practical summary of how autism has the potential to affect individuals' care and treatment

- by pointing out ways in which practice can be made more 'autism sensitive'

- by offering practical strategies and suggestions for practice.

Though this book is primarily addressed to health professionals, I hope that parents, carers, partners, teachers, classroom assistants, social workers, nursery nurses or anyone with an interest in autism (or who has an autism spectrum condition) will also find this short awareness-raising guide accessible and user-friendly and that it may be on hand to help you the next time health needs become an issue.

The key aim of the book is simply this: to emphasise that people with an autism spectrum condition require and deserve special understanding and empathy to help them to understand their world as other people see it. As poor communicators of their own needs and aspirations, like the rest of us they rely on an imperfect system to determine the right kind of health care for them as individuals. Without due consideration of their difficulties in relation to accessing and making sense of health care interventions, it is hard to see how appropriate health services can usefully be evaluated and developed in the future.

Ethically, legally and morally we all have an obligation to share and determine best available practice. As problems are recognised, shared and (it is hoped) documented, fewer mistakes will be made and more people with autism enabled to reach their true potential.

As clinicians respond with clinical audits, risk assessments and practice guidelines, practice will become more 'autism-friendly' and people and families will become more confident and less reluctant to approach health workers for information and advice. General health and well-being should improve as a result. Well, that's my assumption as a former nurse educator and interested parent anyway!

At the end of the book I offer a brief guide to 'fast facts' that health professionals should know about the autism spectrum before caring for or treating the person with autism, together with recommendations for further reading. If you are completely new to the subject of autism, it might be useful to dip into that section now. In the next chapter I go on to make some practical suggestions for managing a visit to the family doctor, as this highlights some of the potential problems of which we should all be aware.

# 2 Consultation and Health Assessment

## Health awareness in people with autism

Beliefs about health and illness are grounded in people's wider understanding of the world in which they live. The stock of knowledge they draw on to 'read' bodily signs of illness owes much to their culture and established norms of behaviour (Radley 1994). If you have a poor conception of your emotional and physical 'selves' and few ways of communicating and sharing your culture, then your stock of available knowledge is likely to be small. The idea of health is also unlikely to mean very much unless you have the language and understanding to question and make sense of it as a concept that has relevance to your needs.

People with autistic spectrum conditions get sick and are vulnerable to the same health problems as everyone else; but, as authors Wainscott and Corbett have advised, they may also have special needs associated with coexisting medical conditions. On top of this, there may be problems related directly to the autism itself, including problems of communication and sensory interpretation (Wainscott and Corbett 1996).

The carer of a person profoundly affected by autism will have learned to recognise the outward signs that all is not well with their relative or client. A child or adult with autism with very limited use of functional language may be unable to express the level of pain or discomfort they are feeling, or make connections between the possible source or reasons for the discomfort being experienced.

All that may alert a parent or carer in the case of a person with poor (or non-existent) language ability is a slight or marked difference in normal routines or behaviour; general outward signs of distress, such as crying, screaming or shouting; restlessness; unexplained agitation; an increase in 'comforting' rituals; or clutching at the actual site of pain. Because these signs can occur on any ordinary day for different reasons it can be hard to distinguish between a minor variation on 'normal' and a real cause for concern.

Carers and parents have to achieve a difficult balance between potentially misinterpreting or misreporting symptoms of apparent illness, and inadvertently neglecting signs or symptoms that might herald illness or an underlying health problem requiring professional attention. Consequently some parents and carers can adopt either a high- or a low-risk approach to potential health problems, with some preferring to err on the side of caution at all times, and others choosing to 'wait and see' in much the same way as any parent or carer does in the conventional family or care setting.

The stakes could be said to be considerably higher in the case of a patient with autism, however, because their ability to convey signs or level of discomfort felt are extremely poor compared with those of the general population, and their sensitivity to pain and other stimuli may be markedly different from the norm. Children and adults who have a history of inappropriate or 'challenging' behaviour (or of self-injury) may also react to pain stimuli and to caring responses in a different way, making an accurate diagnosis and chance of appropriate treatment even harder to achieve.

High levels of anxiety can further complicate the issue, and for people with autism who have difficulty in planning or setting priorities, attention to physical pain or discomfort may not come first on their list. Other things (like adherence to favoured routines or rituals) may take priority over everything else, and where the person is unable to decode bodily sensations effectively enough to register them as pain, serious illness can intervene before appropriate help is sought.

## Going to the doctor

The decision to consult a doctor can depend on many things: how well the patient with autism is able to make themselves understood, how accessible and 'autism-friendly' the doctor is perceived to be, and how confident the parent, carer or patient is that the trip (or visit) will be worth the considerable strain involved in making the consultation in the first place.

Not all people with autism will be able to recognise their shortcomings in communication terms, or to communicate their needs in a way that will endear them to busy health professionals. In a distressed person with Asperger's syndrome, for example, the need to communicate their pain may be asserted loudly with complex over-formal language and with little or no attention being paid to norms of social behaviour (relating their symptoms graphically to everyone in the bus queue, for example, not waiting their 'turn' to be called for consultation in the clinic or interrupting other people's conversations to convey their needs). Because this can (understandably!) be misconstrued as obstructive, bizarre or aggressive behaviour, it can easily distract attention away from the actual physical problems involved, as well as aggravating other people who may be in the vicinity.

People with autism have a very poor sense of other people's thought processes, feelings and intentions towards them (what Simon Baron-Cohen and colleagues have termed 'mindblindness'). It is sometimes difficult, therefore, to convey to them how they can be helped and who the professional 'helpers' might be (for an extended essay on this subject, see Baron-Cohen 1997). You know what you are here for as a health professional, but to the person with autism you may be just another stranger in a strange and very confusing world. Even if you are the regular family doctor or practice nurse, you may not always be recognised by your 'patient' with an autism spectrum disorder unless you are in your 'usual place' (wherever that might be) and adopting behaviour and activities that he or she is familiar with and understands.

Attempts to get 'physical', even within the normally permitted boundaries of health assessment and health care, may therefore be strongly resisted, even when you have successfully attended to or treated the person on a previous occasion. Any 'hands-on' intervention, such as trying to take a pulse or blood pressure reading, dress a wound or assess the nature of an injury, is likely to be rejected unless your patient understands your intentions and has signalled their preparedness to accept your intervention and any necessary discomfort that may be associated with it.

Without sensitive, careful explanation and forewarning of what is to come, your actions may be interpreted at a much more profound level, as an attack or sensory intrusion of some kind, for example, resulting in the possibility of a defensive reaction, such as running away, rocking back and forth, resorting to stereotypical behaviour as an outlet for the distress, or, more difficult still, hitting out at the perceived attacker. The practice of calling colleagues or others in to help in this situation – and perhaps trying to use some form of physical restraint – can compound the problem further. While onlookers see this as a straightforward issue of unwarranted aggression requiring control, the patient with autism may experience a further rush of panic, fear or uncertainty, and have no apparent option but to hit out again if no end to the 'assault' on his or her body appears to be in sight.

Anxious to avoid such a scenario and its consequences from developing, parents and carers can seem fretful or over-protective during a consultation, especially if they take the further risk of antagonising health professionals by suggesting alternative strategies to those being used at the time.

Patients may sometimes make their initial approaches to one of the national telephone advice helplines (NHS Direct in England and Wales, NHS 24 in Scotland). They may then be directed to acute service providers via designated 'primary care centres' (the name given to centres used for the provision of out-of-hours services). If telephone advice is insufficient to help the caller deal with their problem, they can be referred to a GP for an urgent personal consultation, who can then refer on to hospital care. In my experience, even the more able person with autism who lives alone would have considerable trouble negotiating their way through this system without considerable support and guidance. I assume that helpline staff (who are usually trained, experienced nurses) will have sufficient training and insight to recognise that their enquirer has a communication difficulty, although how far this would extend is hard to tell without further systematic examination of real case studies.

I only point to it here as an area that could usefully be explored further and where those supporting people with autism who live alone could help to develop a strategic action plan for use as and when needed.

## Understanding the autistic patient

Concerns expressed by parents and carers point to a lack of knowledge and insight from health workers and professionals as to the nature of autism and the ways in which it affects a person's responses to medical treatment and health care generally. In residential schools support workers have generally developed experience and expertise in dealing with youngsters when they are ill or visiting the doctor, and other health care professionals have learned to listen carefully to their hard-won insights. This is less true where such children are expected to conform in mainstream schooling and to 'fit in' to existing health care systems.

One strategy that health professionals have been known to rely on is that of assuming that people with autism will respond in the same way as 'anyone else with a learning disability'. But people with autism may or may not have an associated learning disability, and those with Asperger's syndrome or high functioning autism may have normal or above-average intelligence and intellectual capabilities. Previous experience of treating people with Down's syndrome, for example, does not necessarily equip health professionals to respond appropriately to the specific needs of the person with autism. Like people who have Down's syndrome (or anyone else, for that matter), people with autism bring a range of attitudes and experiences that are unique to them, and responses that signify their own particular difficulties in relating to the world. They also have shared difficulties that are specific to autism. Acknowledging straight away that the autistic patient's needs may be highly idiosyncratic and individualised puts you, as a clinician or health professional, on much safer ground. Parents and carers will be in a good position to explain just what this means for the individual and the family concerned, and are often able to guide health professionals as to the best course of action given the alternatives available.

Because people with an autistic spectrum condition don't always understand the reciprocal nature of relationships, they are unlikely to see that as health professionals you, too, appreciate an acknowledgement of your help, even if it only extends to observing the normal everyday courtesies of life. Poor or inappropriate eye contact is a common characteristic shared by people with autism. They may find it difficult to talk and look at you at the same time, for example. They may avoid eye contact altogether. Sometimes they will stare inappropriately and this can add to their chances of having their intentions towards others misunderstood.

To be grateful for help, however, is to recognise that you needed it in the first place, and that special skills or attributes were required in order to provide care effectively. The responses of people with autism cannot, by definition, be effusive, and the lack of basic skills of social interaction (as in the appropriate levels of eye contact, smiling, acknowledging receipt of the 'gift' that is care) can make caring or helping someone appear less immediately rewarding. It is only when you have come to recognise the pure joy of 'small victories' in the development of the person who has autism (ask any parent and they will give you an example!) that you recognise how far you have travelled and how much you have achieved in your time together. Communicating with a person who has autism can be a profound learning experience for those who take the time to value its lessons and can teach a great deal about the intricacies of the practitioner–patient relationship.

Novack (1999) has drawn attention to the fact that despite better-constructed basic communication courses in the pre-clinical years, 'medical schools rarely teach and assess students' abilities in the more advanced and subtle skills of communicating with patients in difficult clinical situations' (p.xii). Aware of the urgent need to rectify the present practices of trial and error for many, he encourages professionals to reflect on the different biases, attitudes and values affecting the communication process and to raise their own self-awareness in the interests of developing meaningful practice.

People with autism provide unique opportunities to help health professionals recognise and develop their communication skills, even though their motivation and needs may not be easy to identify. It is possible to develop very positive and helpful strategies that make consultation and health assessment easier, as illustrated later in this chapter.

As a health professional, you can get off to a sound start by first of all acknowledging that parental, carer and individual concerns are usually justified, and by recognising that (in the main) they are likely to relate to the following issues:

- making a decision about whether and when medical or nursing advice is necessary
- managing their own and the patient's anxiety in the meantime
- communicating intentions to the patient (what will happen next and why)
- managing the journey to the consultation (or the wait for a visit)
- making sure the consultation goes smoothly
- encouraging the patient to comply with expectations
- managing any subsequent care or treatment
- minimising the negative effects of illness or worry
- educating the patient to recognise the need to report illness and stay well in the future.

## Key strategies for an effective consultation and health assessment

Four basic strategies can be applied to anyone with an autistic spectrum condition:

- Provide a safe environment.
- Pay close attention to sensory problems.
- Maintain a clear sense of structure.
- Appreciate the family circumstances and history.

### Provide a safe environment

A basic and very reliable tenet is that the person who feels safe will respond much more positively. A lot of what you do as a health professional relates to making your patient feel as safe as possible within the context in which care is being delivered. This requires attention to environmental factors and to issues affecting time and space which will be discussed in more detail below.

Fear and anxiety brought on by any injury or illness is multiplied many times over by the additional problem of not being able to anticipate or understand the process of events involved in a consultation. It should be borne in mind that difficulties in generalising one experience to another can mean that the person is not able to transfer experience or learning from a previous interaction and may have to relearn the process from scratch each time, even when as a practitioner you know the person or family well.

### Pay close attention to sensory problems

This will help to allay the fears of the patient with autism and make it much more likely that your patient will co-operate. To understand the difficulties experienced it is first necessary to understand the processing problems people with autism experience with regard to sensory regulation and making sense of the world they could be said to privately inhabit (discussed in Chapter 1).

Advice on how to prepare for and manage sensory problems will be given in relation to different aspects of care later in the book.

### Maintain a clear sense of structure

Remember that a clear sense of structure, along with positive empathy and a calm, non-judgemental approach, is essential to a successful consultation. Explain clearly what is happening as you go along. Help the person concerned understand by making sure they know what is going to happen next and why. (For example, 'I have to go and find X; I will come back soon – please stay here until I return.') Don't assume the person will know when the consultation has finished. Be clear about what you intend and what the outcomes are intended to be. (One child with autism was asked to hold the door open for some visitors to pass through. He held it for three hours because no one had told him to close it again, and no one had noticed he stayed behind.)

### Appreciate the family circumstances and history

Finally, the family circumstances and history of a person with autism will have had an impact on their attitudes towards professionals in the public services. This could have implications for the success or failure of any advice you give. You might say that this is true of any patient, but as your patient may have a very poor concept of time, referring to 'your last visit' or 'a future appointment' may not mean very much. They may have difficulty in seeing any notion of past or future and may not recall a previous visit or illness. Concentration spans may be short and it may require a great deal of skill and ingenuity to help them focus on what is happening and what needs to be done during the time set aside for the consultation.

In a busy clinic notes may have to be clearly marked so that the attending doctor or nurse will know immediately to modify their normal approach to consultation. Some people carry identification cards outlining their developmental difficulties and asking for clear instructions and tolerance of their lack of social awareness. A brief copy of this can be appended to medical notes or highlighted on the computer records to enable a locum or practitioner who is unfamiliar with autism to recognise that the consultation may not follow the usual pattern.

## A 'safe space' for consultation

### Sensory problems

If at all possible, it is helpful if you can see the person with an autistic spectrum condition at the very beginning or end of surgery or consulting hours, so that if the patient is noisy or unable to comply with expected standards they don't also become the centre of unwanted attention. The more spectators there are around the more likely it is that the person will 'act up'. Children on the spectrum can be extremely sensitive to tensions in the atmosphere and the general 'busyness' of care settings or staff bustling about is likely to increase their 'edginess rating' and encourage signs of uncertainty, such as pacing or shouting. The person with them may become anxious as a result – fearing a scene – and this too will raise the general 'arousal' level of the patient.

Clinical psychologist Teresa Bolick describes the problem as one of 'self-regulation', in that the ability to establish and maintain the level of arousal/alertness, attention, activity and affect (or emotion) appropriate to the situation at hand may be greatly reduced in a person with autism (she describes these as the 'Four As': Bolick 2001). Because arousal levels are directly related to the 'fight or flight' responses of the sympathetic nervous system, any increase in arousal will be accompanied by a release of adrenaline into the body, and an accompanied rise in breathing and heart rates. For the person with autism this can increase their overall levels of excitability and lead them to do one of several things.

They can resort to several learned or instinctive strategies to protect themselves from the uncomfortable feelings this creates; for example, rocking, head-banging or humming. Because such people can suffer from sensory underload (i.e. lack of normal sensitivity to sensations or responses to pain stimuli) or from sensory overload (over-sensitivity to stimuli that would be more easily borne in an individual without autism), they will react very differently, depending on their level of sensory awareness and their particular vulnerabilities at the time.

Lorna Wing (an eminent psychiatrist in the autism field and parent of a daughter with autism) remarks that parents often think their young children with autism may be deaf because they don't react to the kind of loud noises that would send the rest of us running for cover, although they usually realise this isn't the case when the child responds immediately to other sounds, such as a favourite jingle on television or the sound of chocolate being unwrapped. Some sounds will be perceived as intensely distressing (which is why children in class or standing by the roadside will often flinch and cover their ears) while other sounds will be a source of fascination or, alternatively, just be ignored. These may lessen with increasing age and may eventually disappear however (Wing 2001).

In a busy surgery or hospital clinic the background noise of children playing in the toy corner, telephones ringing and people chatting may be enough to instil fear in a person with autism. They can intuitively pick up on the general atmosphere of concern or anxiety in the room, even though they may not be able to articulate the reasons for the anxiety or why people are there in the first place. A hospital casualty department with its bright lights and high level of emotion and activity challenges the senses of most people, but to a person with autism the sensory impact can be intolerable. The urge to run away or to find somewhere calmer can lead them to barge in on or intrude on the privacy of others. Changes to habit and routine present a major difficulty that can't always be assuaged with the normal levels of reassurance offered by health professionals. People with autism often have a very powerful 'need for sameness' (Whitaker 2001).

In much the same way as people with asthma have to be taught the triggers which bring on or exacerbate their asthma symptoms, families and individuals with autism can learn to anticipate the sensory triggers that are likely to cause upset or concern. Remember too that sensory problems can be cumulative and that it may take only a small trigger to send a person who has been struggling for hours or days to adapt to a change into what parents have come to recognise and describe as 'melt-down'.

This is when the vulnerable person becomes overwhelmed by their particular situation and can lash out or indeed hurt themselves by losing control over their emotions and their bodies. This is easier to prevent than to deal with once it has happened, by paying attention to the potential triggers and attempting to avoid or subdue them in some way. Sensory problems in relation to visual stimuli, smells and, above all, touch can render individuals acutely vulnerable, particularly if their ability to make sense of their environment is affected and their ability to perceive people as people and not as 'bags of skin' (as one person with autism has described them) gets in the way of normal self-regulation and reasoning.

Remember, too, that some people with autism will have unusual sensory habits. Lianne Holliday Willey, who has Asperger's syndrome, provides a valuable insider account of this:

> Many a time my actions brought my parents and me to the hospital. I loved to chew crunchy things, even if they were poisonous. When I was finished with my little tin foil table settings, I used to chew them until they crackled their way into a tight, neat ball. I shaved the sand from emery boards with my front teeth. I took great

delight in grinding the striking strip of a matchbook between my back teeth.

I chewed sugar packets whole, loving the way the grainy sweet sugar overcame the bitter paper packet. I ate school paste and play dough and paraffin. I might have avoided the trips to the hospital if I had stopped my grazing there. Unfortunately, I also enjoyed the toilet bowl sanitizing bars and mothballs. My parents tell me people at the hospital began to suspect them of child abuse.

Stiff things, satiny things, scratchy things, things that fit too tightly were all a problem, causing a general sense of unease. Noises and bright lights were almost impossible to bear. High frequencies and brassy, tin sounds clawed my nerves. Whistles, party noisemakers, flutes and trumpets and any close relatives of those sounds disarmed my calm ... Together the sharp sounds and the bright lights were more than enough to overload my senses. My head would feel tight, my stomach would churn, and my pulse would run my heart ragged until I found a safety zone. (Holliday Willey 1999, pp.21–22)[1]

The sensory difficulties some people with an autism spectrum condition experience have been described as 'sensory invasions' (Bolick 2001), a description that is extremely helpful because it conveys the experience from the person's perspective. The message seems to be: Be aware and awake to the possibility of committing or unwittingly causing such an invasion and you will be less likely to get into a meltdown situation.

Much can be done to make the environment feel safe by paying attention to the environment as one of low arousal. A quiet room with no undue disturbances is helpful, as are rooms decorated in neutral colours. The primary colours used to make the children's ward bright and attractive to youngsters, for example, can be visually traumatic for children with autism, particularly as toys and staff uniforms are usually designed with the same themes in mind. Older children and adults may learn to contain their agitation more than younger children, but may still be

1     Excerpt from *Pretending to be Normal: Living with Asperger's Syndrome* (1999) by Liane Holliday Willey reprinted by permission of Jessica Kingsley Publishers, London. © 1999 Liane Holliday Willey.

overcome by their selective receptivity to noise or other distractions (e.g. they may hear the voices of people outside and not be able to distinguish between their voices and yours). Family members or patients themselves may be able to tell you what their triggers are in advance.

Clinical examination is clearly going to be more complicated in a patient who displays 'sensory defensiveness' and who dislikes being touched. People with autism can find the physical closeness of others extremely distressing, which is why they tend to find team or sporting activities very difficult. One young boy who had not been diagnosed with what was later to be described as high functioning autism caused major problems in a school gym hall where he was learning to fence because he couldn't tell the difference between a friendly challenge and an all-out rapier attack. Unable to understand the 'rules' as described by the instructor, he defended himself in the only way he knew how by castigating his perceived attacker and worse.

It is a good idea to keep touch to the minimum wherever possible (even the reassuring handshake or hand on the shoulder can be misinterpreted) and to explain any proposed course of action very clearly.

## Communication

Cognitive or information-processing problems mean that the patient with autism may not be able to take in the advice you give without extra explanation and oodles of reassurance. It helps to write things down and give details to carers or parents if the patient has difficulty reading and this can then be referred to later when the patient is back in more familiar and comfortable surroundings. Remember that patients may be echolalic, that is they may repeat back verbatim things they have heard elsewhere or echo your own questions and advice. This is not intentional and may help them to process information or reduce anxiety, so don't misinterpret this as challenging or disrespectful to you as a person (for advice, see Howlin 1998). Avoid using phrases that can be taken literally. Expressions such as 'crying wolf', 'pull yourself together', 'backs to the wall on this one', 'give me your arm so I can take a blood sample', and 'no need to cry your eyes out' have all caused families real problems in their time!

Teresa Bolick has devised a really useful strategy when communicating with a patient who is becoming distressed or anxious (Bolick 2001).

She describes this strategy as 'low and slow'. Although she is talking about communicating with a teenager, her advice is equally applicable to anyone with autism, although much will depend on their personal level of communication skills. In principle, then,

- keep your eyes below the eye level of your patient and maintain a safe distance (just in case!)

- lower your voice in both volume and pitch

- lower the complexity of your language (don't ask a lot of questions, keep your sentences short and don't preach)

- slow down your own heart rate with slow, deep breaths

- slow down your rate of speech and pause between sentences

- slow down your movements (avoid sudden or threatening movements, move in front of the person rather than behind)

- slow down your agenda and take your time.

Speech and language therapists who specialise in autism are a fount of knowledge on ways in which to improve communication for people with autism. When drawing up local guidelines for treatment, ask them to provide information on visual techniques as many people who have problems communicating their basic needs have acquired skills using pictures or other educational and social resources.

In their *Handbook of Autism* two very experienced speech and language therapists offer a wealth of advice (Aarons and Gittens 1999). It has also been pointed out that as children grow older, their understanding and use of communication and appropriate social behaviour will increase along with their social skills, so that although (for the great majority) they will never 'grow out' of their autism, the condition may become harder to detect in adulthood (Jones, Jordan and Morgan 2001), making the situation for health professionals even more complex.

## If 'meltdown' happens

It is important to stress that there is no inevitable link between autism and challenging behaviour, but that problems are likely to arise when people and the environment fail to satisfy the individual's 'need for sameness'. But what if you have done what you can and meltdown happens anyway?

- Stay calm and in control.

- Never raise your voice.

- Don't crowd or panic your patient (or allow others to).

- Distract if possible.

- Use a favourite toy or known special interests to 'bring down' the patient's level of excitability and restore a sense of calm.

Severely affected people will usually be accompanied to the consultation – but do check how well the carer knows your patient before assuming they know what to do. Try to ascertain what the triggers were for future reference (and note it for others' benefit).

Sedation may very occasionally be needed, but take specialist telephone advice from the duty psychiatrist before doing anything drastic (for information on pharmacological treatments and autism, see also Clarke 1996). Be aware of local policies and any medications already being prescribed.

If security staff or others attempt to stop the person, either by admonishing or physically restraining them, the scene can be set for a major confrontation in which nobody wins. Useful guidelines on the use of physical interventions for staff working with children and adults with a learning disability or autism can be found on the UK Department of Health website (Department of Health 2003a). Advice on the legal issues surrounding the care and control of those presenting with severely challenging behaviour has been drawn up by Professor Christina Lyon of the University of Liverpool and published by the Mental Health Foundation (1994).

## Concluding the consultation

If possible, try to end the consultation on a positive note. Make a note to prepare for next time and discuss with colleagues the possibility of adding some key advice or guidance notes to your patient's records.

Prepare to be surprised each time, however, as no two consultations are likely to be the same, and just because something didn't go right on one occasion, don't assume that this is going to be the template for future consultations.

It's amazing how quickly it is possible to establish a rapport with your patient who has an autism spectrum condition once they have come to recognise your appreciation of their difficulties and anxieties. A sound therapeutic relationship can follow that will impact on the whole family's ability to thrive and flourish, despite the sometimes gloomy predictions about how people are likely to manage aspects of their lives.

People at the more able end of the spectrum could well have been coming to you unrecognised for years – people who may have occasionally puzzled you with the quality and content of their interactions that, at the time, may have seemed a little odd or bizarre. Autism is beginning to explain a good deal of the emotional and behavioural difficulties of people who in the past have been written off as extremely eccentric or rude.

Becoming autism aware can sometimes throw new light on the communication difficulties of so-called 'difficult' patients. As the UK National Autistic Society says, 'the problem is understanding'. As our understanding and experience of helping the person with autism expands, there will no doubt be much more for us all to learn about our relationships with others and not just those with an autism spectrum condition.

# 3 Going to Hospital

All hospitals open for public services should provide 'a staff reasonably sufficient for the foreseeable requirements of the patient', according to Lord Justice Dillon in Bull v. Devon Area Health Authority (1989), a case concerning the organisation of maternity services (see Tingle 1995). People and families affected by autism could therefore be argued as reasonable in requesting any extra help they need to support their loved one who has been admitted to hospital for clinical investigations, care or treatment. From the health care provider's perspective there is also the issue of clinical governance to be considered, whereby staff move from the position of learning from past failures to sharing and spreading good practice (see Donaldson 2000). As England's Chief Medical Officer at the Department of Health, Professor Sir Liam Donaldson provides a healthy dose of pragmatism for practitioners seeking to find out why some health organisations fail while others succeed: 'If you always do what you always did, you will always get what you always got' (Donaldson 2000, p.1).

This wisdom, handed down to him from his astute Scottish granny, rests perfectly with the aims of this book, which is to give practitioners in health and social care the background knowledge to enable them to challenge any existing unhelpful practices and to develop a reliable evidence base for new and more appropriate ones. It is also about giving patients and their supporters the opportunity to ask the relevant questions pertinent to high-quality care.

## Attending hospital as a visitor

To begin with, I'd like to look at the behaviour expected of someone entering a district general hospital as a visitor to see a sick friend or relative. This may be the first time a person with autism experiences this kind of hospital life, and it's a good opportunity to familiarise them with public and staff expectations.

The arrival at the hospital alone can be a daunting experience, particularly if the person with autism is travelling unaccompanied. There may be a range of signposts indicating different departments together with instructions on parking restrictions, instructions for delivery personnel, advice as to where emergencies will be attended to, ambulances parked, and so on.

The entrance to a hospital building is likely to be a busy, confusing place with a plethora of visual and written information pinned up on walls or notice-boards to guide patients, staff and other visitors. Very modern hospitals are often designed to an 'airport' or 'shopping mall' specification, so that it may not obviously be a hospital at all. There may be banks, newspaper and flower stalls and bookshops or pharmacies to be negotiated before an area recognisable as a hospital 'reception area' can be identified. There may be a queue of people already waiting. The lighting may be bright and colourful, with patient information stacked in strategically placed racks or video advice being dispensed from televisions suspended in the corners of waiting areas.

All of this can have a sensory impact on the visitor with autism, and each has the potential to place a demand on them that would otherwise not be thought about by ordinary visitors. The accumulation of visual and auditory stimuli may in themselves be enough to provoke anxiety, especially if other people are in close physical proximity.

The social rules of turn-taking and waiting in line may not be appreciated by the person with autism, and, concentrating on the task in hand, they may approach anyone (remember uniforms and name badges may not mean a lot) for help or information. Their behaviour will seem unconventional to some and perhaps rude or inconsiderate to others. They may not recognise frailty when they see it, and it is quite common for a person with more severe autism to use inappropriate gestures (touching, smelling, pulling at clothes) in order to establish their whereabouts, and perhaps to laugh or grimace at things that (to the more socially aware) appear ill-mannered and distasteful. You may see the elderly person walking slowly with a walking frame or the person hobbling in a plaster cast. You may spot the distraught couple crying in a corner after receiving bad news, or anxiously waiting for news of a loved one. To the person with autism it is the task in hand they are concentrating on (which is getting from A to B), so that little or no acknowledgement may be made of other people or their needs. Unresponsiveness and lack of attention to other people is a recognised feature of autism spectrum conditions (see Baron-Cohen and Bolton 1993).

If they are unable to communicate their needs with language sufficiently well to be understood, physical gestures may be used in order to gain attention. Sometimes personal identification will be carried giving an indication of the person's difficulties. However he or she presents, it may take considerable tact and sensitivity to verbal and non-verbal cues to elicit the kind of help or guidance your visitor needs. Facial expression may be passive and 'wooden' in the person with autism. It may be hard to gauge what the person is thinking. They may appear to 'look right through you' when spoken to or challenged.

Staff working in the reception areas of hospitals should be alerted to the behaviours and needs of people with autism to a point where they can at least identify characteristic behaviours. This would reduce the potential for misunderstandings and altercations, as well as saving time and unnecessary distress for everyone involved. My own local hospital has an informal reception desk attended by representatives of the hospital's League of Friends. Usually mature volunteers, they are there to welcome patients and visitors and to direct or accompany them to where they need to go. This can save paid staff considerable time and also give the hospital a more friendly, sociable atmosphere. They too can be prepared for the person who lacks confidence and can do much to make the experience calmer and less stressful by listening and attending carefully to their visitor's requests.

It's worth remembering that in an autistic condition the pitch and volume of a person's voice may also be affected. They may appear to shout or gesticulate rudely as a result. Alternatively the person may talk in a flat, low monotone without the characteristic inflections of the average voice. This doesn't necessarily indicate depression or a lack of interest, it may just be their normal way of expressing themselves. Many parents have wished for a 'volume control' button for their children, since being talked to loudly for long periods can be very wearing. It may be very difficult for the person affected to modulate the voice, however, and you should never respond by shouting back or talking equally loudly or you may make the situation worse. A gentle reminder that your ears are hurting may be enough.

Having arrived at the ward they wish to visit, again there may be written instructions as to visiting arrangements and time restrictions. At this point it is worth remembering the tendency to take things literally experienced by many people with autism. One very able man I know with autism encountered the sign 'Fire Door – Keep Shut'. The problem was that he needed to get to the other side of the door. So what did he do? Whom did he ask? No one. He simply gave up and went home again. The sign said 'Keep Shut' after all, so he did exactly as he had been instructed.

If waiting times are restricted, he or she may not know that the rules are sometimes used flexibly for close relatives, visitors who have travelled a long distance or those who have been unavoidably delayed. It may say that the ward closes at 4pm but what if it is now 4.05pm? One important aspect of autism is supreme difficulty in being flexible about routines. People affected will often be rule-bound and extremely rigid in their thinking.

When greeting your visitor you should identify yourself and guide them directly to where they want to go, at the same time pointing out who to ask if they have any other worries and concerns.

The design of hospitals and ward or departmental layout may mean that they will be close to other patients and within hearing distance of their private conversations. It may be helpful here to point out where the accepted boundaries are, the normal practice regarding toilet facilities or waiting rooms, any procedures in force restricting contact with infectious patients, and which furniture can be used. Personal or hospital belongings may also have to be explained so that your visitor doesn't inadvertently help himself or herself to other people's private property.

Routines for protecting patients against cross-infection, such as hand-washing, should also be explained (although being instructed to

'Wash your hands in the toilet over there' might literally be interpreted as washing hands in the toilet bowl, so again be careful with your language). Echolalia can mean that overheard conversations may be stored and repeated indiscriminately (and perhaps loudly) elsewhere, so care and tact will be needed to avoid this.

You will also need to prepare your visitor for any unexpected sights, smells and sounds, such as bleeping monitors, blood transfusions, specialised equipment, the rattle of dinner trolleys and the constant ringing of hospital telephones. He or she may not understand the need for patients to rest and may expect the person being visited to do all their usual things.

Being confined to bed or having 'no-go' areas (e.g. wounds, dressings, ventilators, heart monitors, traction trolleys, intravenous drips, catheter bags and surgical drainage equipment) may puzzle your visitor. Shiny equipment or things that can be pulled, twiddled and played with may hold a fascination for those with strong sensory compulsions.

It may also be difficult for the person to sit quietly, because there may be an element of hyperactivity associated with their neurological impairment. You will need to use your discretion and any available information regarding your visitor's sensibilities to ascertain what to do for the best in a given situation. The person they are visiting may be able to offer you some valuable insight and clues.

This is perhaps a good time to raise two important caveats. Some people assume that because of their disability, people with autism don't feel emotions in the same way as other people, and they sometimes go so far as to assume that they therefore don't care what happens to those closest to them. Some also confuse level of verbal ability with level of understanding. When breaking bad news to a relative with autism or conveying a concern, don't be tempted (as in past generations) to assume either that they are uninterested or that they won't have an opinion to offer or concerns to discuss.

Even those people with little or no language may be able to communicate in pictures or by signing. Those with language (and especially those with high functioning autism) may, in contrast, demonstrate very sophisticated language. They may recall and be minutely aware of aspects of care or the nature of a particular condition, and may talk about it at length. Remember, too, that a proportion of people with autism will have normal or above-average intelligence (as defined by standard IQ tests). You will therefore have to exercise judgement as to the language you use to discuss any concerns or questions they may have.

Observe the person carefully for different indicators of psychological distress such as general agitation, rocking or 'crooning' or banging fists against walls, as well as the more obvious signs of tearfulness or repeating the same phrases over and over again.

Find out whether the person is known to social services – there may be someone familiar with the person and their everyday behaviour who may be available to 'mediate' and advise. Don't hesitate to call on colleagues with more direct experience in autism, such as nursing, medical or psychologist colleagues in community-based learning disability or mental health services.

Voluntary sector advocacy organisations for service users and carers and the websites of national organisations that specialise in autism offer a range of services from factsheets to workshops and telephone helplines. They also produce material for health and social care professionals which is inexpensive and easy to obtain (see Appendix 2).

More will be conveyed about bereavement and autism later in the book, but it is worth pointing out at this stage that people with autism, and particularly those with learning disabilities, have been the recipients of poor care in the past when it was assumed (wrongly) that they were unable to understand issues such as serious illness and death. Remember also that attachment to objects and places can be as acute for people with autism as attachment to those people closest to them. They need as much advance warning as possible to any change in routine, or any changes to their normal surroundings. The potential loss of someone close requires careful handling in the same way as any other change in their lives. The adaptation process may be lengthy and complex and may be greeted initially with shock and protest. However, it isn't possible to generalise about the kinds of loss that will elicit the greatest reaction, as each individual will have their own idiosyncratic attachments to objects, people, personal places, and so on (see Morgan 1996).

## Attending hospital clinics

Hospital outpatient departments are generally busy, overcrowded places that rely heavily for success on patients being extremely 'patient' and carefully observing the informal social rules that have evolved over time. When referring patients with autism for a formal specialist consultation it is helpful to inform the specialist of any special needs or anxieties the patient may have prior to attending for the appointment. There is of course the issue of confidentiality to be considered – not every person with an autistic condition will wish their autism diagnosis to be made known. As autism is generally accepted as a medical diagnosis, it would seem to be in the person's best interests to have whatever additional health problem they are experiencing assessed in the context of their existing disability, so that most referring physicians or health practitioners would include this information in the referring letter or documentation. Not all patients with autism welcome this, however, and some parents have difficulty in ever accepting the autism diagnosis, making the issue more complex for some doctors.

If the patient with autism is living in supported residential accommodation or in a specialist boarding school, their care is the primary responsibility of the establishment concerned. The person will usually be accompanied by their key worker who is there to support him or her during the consultation process.

While family involvement is strongly encouraged in most residential settings, not all parents wish (or are able) to be fully involved in sharing decisions about their relative. Sometimes it is the extended family who prefer to be consulted. For those people with more profound autism, adoptive or foster carers may be involved. Care may be shared between natural parents and regular respite carers.

Adults with autism may live independently and act autonomously or may be accompanied by a partner or spouse. Adults who have never left the family home may be accompanied by a parent or by a representative of the family from one of the voluntary organisations (such as carers' associations or citizen advocacy schemes).

Whatever the home situation, it will help the doctor being consulted if the situation can be explained either before or early on in the consultation so that everyone is clear about the practicalities of who is sharing in decision-making and whose wishes need to be taken into account. This can prevent serious misunderstandings and can provide the important link with home that may be needed to ensure health care needs are met.

From the patient's perspective several aspects will need to be managed carefully:

- reminding the patient of the need for the appointment and explaining the necessary disruption to normal routine involved

- remembering the appointment and making the necessary arrangements

- making the journey to and from the clinic

- managing the wait to be seen (especially if the clinic is busy)

- handling the consultation itself (together with any tests or clinical observations involved, e.g. history-taking, urine tests, weight measurement, physical examination, attending for X-rays)

- making sure your patient understands and consents to any treatment (or appropriate parental/carer consents are obtained)

- recognising and making contingency plans for any known sensory 'triggers', fears or anxieties that may provoke an unhelpful behavioural reaction

- ending the consultation with a clear idea of any further health care intervention that may be necessary and of whether any further advice or information is required to support the person through whatever is planned.

This may seem to be rather an onerous list, but parents and people with autism who have experienced the health care system know only too well that failure to take all of the above into account can lead to real difficulties.

Parents have been labelled as difficult and obstructive for trying to explain why precautions may have to be put in place. Where such advice has been ignored or dismissed, not only do the people involved feel devalued, but the quality of care is put at risk, with the added possibility that behavioural reactions can lead to a loss of control. The main ingredient in any unwanted reaction is likely to be fear and anxiety. By planning to reduce that anxiety the chances of a successful consultation are far greater. There are several very practical things that the doctor or health professional being consulted can do to minimise risk. These include:

- asking parents/carers or the person concerned to devise a sensory profile of your patient so that you can minimise and address any sensory triggers

- making appointments at a time when the clinic is relatively quiet (over lunch, at the very beginning or end of the day)

- explaining who you are and what you have been asked to do

- making sure your patient isn't hungry or over-tired

- using any special interests your patient may have to help them feel at ease (these include obsessive interests of all sorts from ants to train timetables, fascination with numbers, or a special toy)

- recognising when you are beginning to get into difficulty (being sensitive to small physiological changes that can herald a problem, such as signs of general agitation, increase in heart rate and respiration, flaring of nostrils, grunting, rocking and pacing).

It is, of course, always important to listen carefully to what patients themselves 'say'. If they are unable to communicate clearly through language, examine their behaviour as a communicative act – if the behaviour could speak, what would it say? ('No, that hurts!' 'Who are you?' 'Where am I?') It is better to withdraw quietly and try again later than pursue an action regardless of its possible consequences.

It is worthwhile to attend to any strategies offered by parents, carers or key workers, provided you consider them reasonable in the circumstances. Most families have devised their own tried and tested strategies for managing their relative's difficulties, but not all may seem strictly ethical to those with no experience! Advice may be needed from a clinical psychologist or consultant psychiatrist with expert knowledge in autism.

Colleagues in the community psychiatric nursing or learning disability service are also usually able to provide guidance and advice.

Remember to allow for any additional learning disability or coexisting health problem, and don't forget that although autism is neither a mental illness nor a learning disability in itself, anyone with an autism spectrum condition may have an additional mental health problem or an additional learning disability.

Sorry to labour the point, but do pay attention to the language you use. One family doctor I know asked a young patient with autism to 'punch him on the nose if his special skin treatment didn't work'. I think you can probably guess what happened...

Be aware that your patient may not process the information you give them in the usual way. They may hear or take in only a fraction of what you say (or focus on particular words or phrases). Always check for understanding and, if you can, ask another appropriate person to make a second check to be as certain as you can that you have communicated effectively. Provide appropriate written or pictorial communications or clarifications, together with an indication of where your patient can go for information if they should forget or have further questions. This will usually, but not always, be the family doctor.

Make sure carers and key workers are also clear about any action they are to take on their relative or client's behalf. And, of course, keep a clear and careful record of the consultation, together with any recommendations for action, whether medical or administrative.

Finally, within the bounds of patient confidentiality and respect for persons, try to use your clinical experiences of the patient with autism as a training opportunity for colleagues who are unfamiliar with the problems experienced. Use both positive and negative experiences as material for 'critical incident analyses' and see what can be added to any existing guidelines your employer may use to help people with autism.

## Attending hospital as an emergency

Many parents' greatest dread is having their child or adult relative have to attend accident or emergency rooms as a casualty. If it becomes necessary, presumably because of an accident, acute illness or ingestion of poisonous substances, they will probably have rehearsed this moment (at least mentally) and be both distressed and concerned that staff will know enough about autism to make themselves understood and to be able to distinguish between 'real' aggression and any distress or agitation that may be induced in their loved one by illness or anxiety.

Adults with autism who find themselves in need of emergency help may not have a diagnosis, or may not appreciate the true nature of their difficulties. Some may well have been excluded from society as a result (see Introduction).

There are several reasons why people with autism might be more likely to attend casualty than the general population. Some of the main factors are:

- a tendency to be accident prone (through inefficient sensory processing or taking instructions literally)

- unusual sensory habits, sensitivities or phobias (e.g. inhalation or ingestion of dangerous or unusual substances, smearing of their own faeces leading to infection)

- ritualistic and sometimes harmful behaviour (such as self-injury, head-banging, biting)

- getting into arguments through rigid and inflexible thinking, and perhaps becoming involved in fights

- responding to touch inappropriately and lashing out at a perceived assailant

- social and sexual naivety leading to inappropriate sexual behaviour and a corresponding vulnerability to sexual, psychological or physical abuse

- vulnerability to neglect or physical abuse where families are not able to cope with their relative's behaviour

- high incidence of epilepsy (about 30 per cent of people with an autism spectrum condition are prone to epileptic seizures).

Emergency health workers understandably focus on the problem being experienced by the person brought to the emergency department and may ask carers or relatives to wait elsewhere while emergency care is given. This is perfectly acceptable in normal circumstances, but in autism it can be disastrous as valuable 'insider' information and interpretation of the patient's behaviour may be needed sooner rather than later.

All of the information given earlier in the book is relevant here. You need to get as much information as possible about the nature of the person's autism, any associated learning disability, linguistic capability and usual patterns of behaviour. People with an autism diagnosis who attend the emergency room unaccompanied may carry identification and an emergency contact number.

Remember that verbal responses from the person with autism may be delayed or unobtainable. You may have to interpret behavioural responses instead.

Give them time to respond and orientate themselves. Bear in mind that some may present with problems allied to their neurological vulnerability. The usual baseline you use for observations of vital signs may not cover every possibility (e.g. catatonia). Look again at some of the issues raised above and ask yourself whether any of them are relevant to your patient. Inability to communicate could be due to a new brain injury as a result of an accident or infection, or because of congenital or acquired brain injury earlier in life.

Be especially sensitive to sensory intrusions (try to reduce noise and bright lights) and, if possible, attend to their needs in a quiet place away from other people.

Take care not to startle the person and don't be surprised if they appear restless and defensive. They may not have the ability to deduce where they are and what is happening for cognitive reasons due to their disability as well as from the effects of illness or accident that brought them to the department in the first place. Care will be needed to differentiate between acute physiological reasons for their clinical presentation and the kinds of behaviour presented because of their difficulty in making sense of their current experience and situation. I can't emphasise enough the importance of having someone experienced stay with your patient at all times. This is not a job for a junior member of staff. Never leave the patient unattended in a cubicle or on a hospital trolley for example, or close to other critically ill patients.

Physical handling should be as gentle as possible and kept to the minimum necessary for successful treatment. Take precautions for your own and others' physical safety. Speak clearly and quietly using direct and uncomplicated language; explain carefully who you are, what you are doing and why; check regularly for understanding. Use 'comforters' or distractors where they are obvious or where you have been alerted to them even if they appear rather odd and eccentric. Keep your body language restrained (don't gesticulate or use expressive gestures). Be aware that you may meet a significant challenge to your efforts. Keep physical restraint to an absolute minimum as this tends to compound problems and increase fear and anxiety.

Some people with autism take medication that might confuse the clinical picture or that could be contributing to their presenting condition (major tranquillisers and jaundice, for example).

Eye contact may seem avoidant or aggressive in the patient with autism, and they may constantly seek reassurance. This is unintentional and doesn't normally imply a wish to harm, although fear may cause them to react physically. A patient may follow you or touch you inappropriately. Be clear in your instructions as to what is acceptable, and above all try to keep your interventions low-key.

If the department has a policy on helping with patients with autism, follow it as far as possible and as seems consistent with his or her situation and presentation. If there is no policy, make sure you set up a small working party afterwards and get the appropriate advice for next time.

Be aware that one of the key problems experienced by people with autism is a failure to understand and decode facial expressions, gestures and body language. They may equally well have difficulty in using situation-appropriate gestures themselves (hence inappropriate giggling or laughter in a serious or grave situation). Your usual reassuring smile may not be enough to calm them if they are feeling bewildered and unsure of what you expect from them.

It is not unusual for patients with autism to present in casualty with several undiagnosed problems because they have not been able to communicate physical or emotional problems earlier in life. If possible, liaise with health and social care professionals in the community to obtain services for your patient if you are discharging them home, and make sure as far as possible that parents and carers are kept informed. Remember that conflicts may occasionally arise between what the patient wants and what parents or carers can cope with. Try to hear all sides of the problem.

Respect confidentiality in the usual way and don't forget (as many, I'm afraid, do) to ask the patient what he or she would like to happen. People with autism – both able and less able – should have their autonomy respected as a matter of course. It is important not to write them off as incapable of sharing in decision-making but to help them participate as far as possible in care decisions. Their expressed priorities may seem odd or strange to you, but remember that any change in routine or circumstances may cause acute distress to the person concerned and may actually cause them more worry than a pressing medical or health concern.

Problems with what psychologists call 'executive functioning' may make it difficult for them to understand or envisage what the implications of a particular illness or situation are for them personally (for a description of executive functioning, see Happe 1994). In lay terms, the problem is a difficulty in prioritising and forward-planning skills that can compromise the person's ability to self-care.

Individualise care as much as possible and, if your patient is to be admitted to hospital, make sure at handover that as much information about the person's difficulties or sensitivities as possible is shared with ward or departmental staff (including anyone involved in diagnostic procedures, such as radiographers, or in transportation, such as porters and ambulance drivers).

If your patient is unconscious, staff will need to have some idea of what to expect when he or she wakes up. Their patient will probably be very disorientated and alarmed. Constant supervision is necessary even if they appear to be awake and co-operative. Your patient may react unpredictably in response to an unexpected or unanticipated stressor and may behave impulsively as a result, putting themselves and others at risk.

When engaging in physical examination or investigation procedures or employing the usual measures to restore physiological homeostasis (such as fluid infusions, blood transfusions), be aware that your patient may not be able to resist tampering with them and observe them carefully for any potential reactions – both physical and behavioural. History-taking will need to be painstaking, and attention will have to be given to avoiding literalism and figures of speech that can be misunderstood. The question 'Do you hear voices?', for example, would probably be met with a simple affirmative. The patient hears your voice or that of the person on the other side of the curtain. It doesn't necessarily mean he or she is psychotic. Try to minimise background noise and distractions and see whether your patient can be helped by deep breathing and relaxation exercises. Try to 'tune in' with your patient's prevailing anxiety (Nally and Bliss 2000).

Try as far as you can to establish trust with your patient, even if a rapport is difficult because of their social and communication difficulties or because of their presenting clinical condition. Prioritise what is important clinically and what can wait until extra support arrives, in the form of, it is hoped, knowledgeable carers or relatives.

I will come on shortly to issues surrounding informed consent to medical procedures and health interventions. If this is likely to be an issue for you now, go to Chapter 4.

Occasionally you may find that it is the relative of the person receiving emergency attention who presents with features of autism. This may appear as extreme anxiety or pedantry (rigid and inflexible thinking). If you should encounter someone who is angry and difficult to reassure or console, consider this as a possibility. Bear undiagnosed autism in mind if someone is difficult to help or if they are exhibiting depressive symptoms and their behaviour seems ritualistic and stereotyped.

When you encounter situations where patients refuse treatment or become inexplicably distressed out of all proportion to their presenting medical problem, keep the autism perspective in mind. Sensory defensiveness is also common for a variety of reasons in people who don't have autism, so care taken to minimise problems of this kind will still be welcome.

Staff working in emergency rooms should be aware of the dangers of jumping to erroneous conclusions and should also learn to recognise the difference between a person who is a 'frequent attender' because of abuse and the person who has sensory compulsions or behavioural difficulties that greatly increase their level of risk, particularly in relation to self-injury and sexual abuse and manipulation. I can't pretend that this will be easy. Those responsible for child and adult protection need to study such risk in more detail so that appropriate recommendations can be made (see the Department of Health draft guidance, 2003b). Autism and sexuality is an area fraught with risk, but guidance and advice is available from the national autistic societies (see Appendix 2).

Another practical issue to consider is that not all people with autism will have the ability to manage their personal hygiene. Even the basics of toileting and controlling bodily functions may present difficulties. Much of the stress that parents experience comes from their children's prolonged dependence on them: they may be unable to eat without help, toilet, dress or wash independently, and this places extreme demands on parental time and energy, as well as being a source of embarrassment to them (Schopler 1995; see also Gillberg 2002). This again is related to their difficulties of organisation and planning, and of 'proprioception' (the ability to 'locate' your body parts in relation to the space around you).

This problem is also commonly seen in patients with acquired brain injury, such as severe head injury or stroke, so that, for example, he or she may wash the top and sides of the face or hair, but not show any awareness of the back of the head. Successful toileting programmes have to teach self-care skills by breaking them down into discrete elements so that each part of the normally taken-for-granted activity is labelled and skills learned by rote. While this is often helpful it can mean that the person is still not able to appreciate the external or environmental aspects of the act, which is to take account of timing and surroundings.

Inappropriate voiding or public exposure of parts of the body normally kept private can result because of the inability to generalise a social rule to a new social situation (toilet doors may not be closed, leading to misunderstandings, clothing may not be adjusted properly, wetting or soiling can occur without warning). Such a lack of self-awareness can understandably cause consternation in public places. Staff working in the emergency department will therefore have to be aware of this potential problem and take averting action.

Sometimes the person will have a fear or phobia of objects or situations that prevent him or her from doing what is necessary. Bear this in mind when undertaking physical procedures or trying to obtain blood or urine samples.

Never assume that patients with autism will know how to collect a urine sample, for example. The planning skills involved may be a major challenge. And don't expect them to know that the blood being taken for analysis is limited to a mere phial's worth. They may assume, as I know one lady with autism did, that you want all the blood they have. One patient who was asked to 'give' a junior doctor her arm so that a blood sample could be collected was left feeling confused and alarmed. She was really rather attached to her arm and expressed an understandable wish to keep it!

## Admission to hospital for investigations or day surgery

Admission to hospital is an anxious time for most people, regardless of their background or domestic situation. The feeling of helplessness and lack of personal control that follows from having to place complete trust in health professionals is a heady mixture, particularly if serious illness is suspected and family income threatened by any proposed change in social circumstances. Communication difficulties add to the risk that needs will be misunderstood. All the people involved make assumptions about the patient and their circumstances, and care and treatment can be affected as a result.

Even where professional values and care appear outwardly excellent, the working 'sub-cultures' operating informally in a health or social care setting can jeopardise care quality, so that some patients receive a higher quality of care than others. Such practices aren't always explicit or even recognised, but they do exist, or we wouldn't have the many abuses exposed in the press and through the policy literature that has been published over the years. Patients can be informally 'labelled' as difficult to deal with. This may be because they are perceived as 'too demanding' or undeserving of care because of personal habits and lifestyle. People with psychological problems in particular require a lot of extra time and reassurance from staff and where emotional problems and negativity have become habitual, this can challenge the patience of health professionals who have many competing demands on their time.

However, one lady with high functioning autism I know prepares for hospital by writing her own care plan and putting the necessary observation charts in order. Because she has to return regularly for treatment, the staff provide her with the requisite forms and information in advance at pre-admission clinics. This has become rather a ritual, but an extremely helpful and necessary one, as it helps her to feel calm about the prospect of admission and treatment and considerably lessens associated anxiety. It's also rather handy for staff who haven't met her before when she attends for treatment! They work on it together so that it is as up to date and as relevant as possible to prevailing concerns.

### Preparing for admission

If a patient has poor social skills and can't communicate needs and wishes, who is going to anticipate their needs? How is effective care going to be planned? In the case of people attending as day patients there is very little time available to explain one's difficulties and avoid misunderstandings, especially if the patient list is long and staff in short supply. The following list of questions to ask yourself isn't exhaustive but it should provide useful pointers for staff working in day units.

- Who has planned the visit and has the patient been properly prepared?

- Has the carer decided to 'leave it to the last minute' for fear of upsetting their relative or client? If so, who is going to break the news, when is this to happen and how will staff know how to respond?

- If the patient has been prepared, are there any immediate issues to be addressed, such as finding 'safe space' privacy or obtaining consent to treatment?

- Have you checked that the patient knows what is to happen and put provision in place for dealing with any unexpected outcomes or surprises?

- Does the patient have any sensory sensitivities that might compromise the necessary access to his or her body for medical investigation and examination? Have strategies been devised for minimising problems?

- What is the patient's usual form of communication? Do staff need to make any special provision in advance?

- Have appropriate transport arrangements been made? Many people with autism will need to be accompanied throughout their journey and their stay in hospital.

- Has a member of staff been allocated special responsibility to observe the patient at all times?

- Has anyone considered conducting a risk assessment before the patient arrives?

- If your patient is likely to be unable to control some bodily functions or aspects of their behaviour, how might this impact on the care of others and the normal running of the unit?

- Has an experienced anaesthetist or pain clinic specialist been consulted regarding any necessary modification to aspects of pain management?

When preparing your patient for clinical investigation, much will depend on the type of referral (i.e. emergency or planned admission). Because of the difficulties in expressing pain or discomfort, it is likely that many people with autism have health problems that only come to professional attention when they are serious or life-threatening, or when those close to them have sensed that something is amiss.

Once formal hospital admission is arranged, the ideal is for the patient to attend a pre-admission clinic where careful explanation and listening to the patient and carers can elicit any worries or preconceptions they may have about care and about the nature of the particular investigation planned. Given the advanced technology available to 21st-century physicians and surgeons, investigations can be quite complex and require different types of co-operation from the person undergoing them.

If someone is familiar with hospitals and their ways of working it is possible for them to anticipate the things that will be done to them and to envisage how they might go about coping. If they have no concept of hospitals or health professionals and very poor planning abilities, this kind of mental rehearsal and self-preparation is unavailable to them. Because they can't anticipate, they can't devise a coping strategy or indeed recognise when what is being done to them is going to end. And if they hear only parts of what they are being told and additionally don't understand the words being used, they are likely to become confused and

panicky and want to escape the situation at the first opportunity. Therefore, before expecting your patient with autism to participate, you will
have to work out an individualised plan of care that takes into account
any identifiable fears, sensory problems or special requests made by the
patient. If he or she is a child or young person, parents or carers may be
available to assist with this.

The person with autism is likely to be very wary of you, so that once
you have explained what is to happen you will need to guide them
through each stage of the process as described. Most people with autism
respond well to any kind of imposed structure, so that a carefully set out
'plan' will help them to adjust to what is being expected of them. Any
deviation from the process outlined is, however, likely to cause some
distress (for example, porters or medical staff not arriving at the expected
time). It would be helpful if staff who are working with the patient are
advised of the situation and the need to be calm and take things at a
steady pace. Talking 'over' the patient is to be avoided as they may misun-
derstand or become very frightened by what they hear and react accordingly.

The atmosphere should be one of 'low arousal' with a minimum of
noise and distraction. My own experience of hospitals would suggest this
could be difficult as the bright lights and bustle of the clinical environment that supports staff in being able to have a (very necessary!) clear
view of what they are doing is rather the opposite of the neutral, low key
and quiet environment that is best for reassuring a person with autism.
Again, physical contact should be kept to the minimum (unless the
patient specifically seems to welcome some kind of 'comforting' contact),
and a member of staff should be allocated to stay with the patient
throughout the procedure and during the period of recovery.

Other people who know your patient well may be able to alert you to
any early signs that the person is becoming agitated, although these will
have to be assessed in the context of the particular investigation being
carried out. Signs of agitation might resemble potential side-effects of the
investigation being carried out, so care will be needed to distinguish
between the two. It is of course also possible to experience the two
together, as allergic or other abnormal responses could well make the
person feel anxious and unwell.

The ability to co-operate with instructions sufficiently to complete the investigation may also be compromised, and some ingenuity might be necessary to ensure that patients comply. (One suggestion made to me is to ask the patient to mimic the actions of the member of staff accompanying them; for example, 'Breathe in like this. Now stop!' when a patient is being X-rayed.) Although this strategy is unlikely to work with more sophisticated procedures, the idea of using autism's facility for mimicry would appear to have potential and could be explored in advance if appropriate to the situation. Actions could be rehearsed and practised several times in advance of the procedure, which may have the added benefit of reassuring the patient at the same time.

## Managing the patient

Be aware that some of the practices commonly adopted for patients (such as inserting a cannula into a vein) should not be attempted on the basis of 'one small scratch and it will be over'. This is unlikely to apply in the patient with autism unless you have been very successful in diverting their attention elsewhere at the time.

Pain may be felt acutely and co-operation withdrawn. Conversely, the person may appear to have little reaction to what to most people would seem quite painful. But a person who seems either impervious to or hypersensitive to pain in one situation will not necessarily react in the same way the next time. 'Selective receptivity' may mean that the person responds to something else in the environment instead. Pain reaction may also be delayed or may be perceived in another part of the body.

Anaesthetists will be able to advise on the right kind of analgesia or sedation for the patient but should have a full clinical history of the patient beforehand and be aware of the specific autism spectrum condition the person has. Many patients require close supervision by anaesthetists or specialist nursing staff particularly where there is a history of epilepsy or other neurological problems.

Clearly the clinical management for a person with classic autism who may be severely withdrawn and uncommunicative will be very different than that for the person with attention deficit hyperactivity disorder who may be able to tell you what they are feeling but have difficulty in concentrating long enough to allow the investigation to take place. Very intrusive investigations such as different forms of endoscopy (anything involving tubes and lights!) will meet with variable responses. Some people with autism may be fascinated by the procedure provided they suffer no discomfort; others will deliver a blanket refusal. Information-giving will be a challenge for staff in these situations – and unfortunately until autism-specific guidelines are drawn up and systematically researched by practitioners, it is hard to suggest any hard and fast rules that are likely to meet with success. If you have read through the previous chapters you will have an idea of the kinds of problems likely to be experienced and will at least be in a position to anticipate them, rather than dealing with them on an ad-hoc basis, as has generally been the position for many people up until now. The more complex or intimate the procedure being undertaken, the more time and care will be needed to devise an acceptable management strategy.

Where problems do arise it is important to communicate events to other staff and to record them accurately in care plans and other patient records. The language used should be clear and explicit and not fall into the trap of making value judgements about the patient (or family and carers) concerned. Informal labelling can do much to harm the patient (however unwittingly) and any aggression experienced should be recognised and dealt with appropriately rather than using the 'red card' or 'yellow card' sometimes favoured by hospitals with policies aimed at reducing assaults on staff. People with autism will not be calmed by such measures, only confused and disorientated further, as they are unlikely to make the abstract connections between hospitals and football necessary to understand your message. Most people with autism think very concretely, and problems can often be traced to literal misunderstandings. One man with undiagnosed autism refused a bowel X-ray because he thought his bowels were literally going to be 'rinsed away' (see Gillberg 2002). This demonstrates how profound the communication difficulty is and how aware we should be of the language we use in caring for people with autism-related problems.

Don't leave equipment or other material around that can be a potential danger to the patient from swallowing or other inappropriate use. Be as gentle and unobtrusive as you can and 'listen' carefully to what their behaviour and reactions tell you in relation to any fears. If parents or carers suggest a strategy, even if it appears time-consuming and 'over the top', listen to it and see whether it or a compromise is acceptable.

Be prepared for the possibility of severe allergic reactions or anaphylaxis as in normal practice, and have an 'action stations' plan for any departure from the usual run of things.

Where special technology is used or injections have to be given (such as endoscopes, 'imaging scanners', X-rays, ultrasound equipment, radio-active dyes) have your patient accompanied and supervised at all times. Bear in mind the need for a safe environment (as described in Chapter 2). However, don't use this as a reason to 'hide' or exclude the patient from normal social contact. Try to be sensitive to their feelings even if it isn't clear what their feelings are from their behaviour. Remember that parents, carers and supporters will also be anxious and apprehensive. You will need to maintain close contact with them.

Again, be aware that any variation in normal routine or surroundings may well cause your patient extreme anxiety especially if an overnight stay is involved. Find out whether anything can be done to mitigate this, either by using the patient's special interests to fill in any waiting time or by bringing in familiar or favoured items from home. Anxiety reactions will sometimes take the form of ritualistic behaviours (running on tiptoes, flapping hands, twirling string, pulling or pushing a toy or piece of furni-ture, rocking or pacing). You will need to take care that any behaviours are kept to safe limits. The more able patient with autism may appear very tense and watchful and talk at length about any worries. That's why having someone confident and experienced to stay with the patient for reassurance is so important. Minimising the time spent in hospital may also help, provided there is informed practical help and support available at home.

If sedation is necessary for any part of a medical investigation, explain what you are doing with care and don't surprise your patient or force them physically. (See also the section on preparing for surgery later in this chapter.) Be particularly aware of the possibility of existing medications and pre-existing medical conditions, allergies or tendency to seizures. I know of one family who pleaded with the radiographer planning an MRI scan to sedate their daughter prior to going into the scanner as she would be unable to understand or stay still as required. This was refused for the

best of reasons (from the professional's perspective) and the patient consequently was unable to tolerate the test. Another appointment had to be
made and due sedation given before the MRI scan could be successfully
completed. Unnecessary anxiety and distress was caused and an extra and
traumatic journey was also required. A much-needed appointment was
lost to the system and the confidence of everyone concerned severely
dented.

Remember that the experience of a short stay may have an enormous
impact on any consequent stays in hospital and could affect the potential
to treat your patient in the future. Traumatic experiences often stay with
the person, even if others didn't recognise the nature of the trauma at the
time. One adult with Asperger's syndrome that I know was involved in a
minor car accident in which no one was physically hurt, but he spent the
next six months or so after the accident repeating 'car banged dead' and
becoming visibly tearful and distressed many times in a day.

Try to gauge the emotional maturity of your 'short-stay' patient and
provide them with mementos or information concerning their stay that
may help them to anticipate and cope with future visits.

Avoid infantilising behaviour or treating adults in a childish way even
if they don't appear to have the intellectual capacity to deal with adult
concepts. Their experience may be a jumble of events that they find difficult to make sense of and interpret.

The more people involved in delivering care, the harder still your
patients may find it to orientate themselves. See if you can tune in to what
they appear to be experiencing and take your lead from there. Consis-
tency and attention to detail is vital.

## Communicating results

Communicating the results of clinical investigations should also be carefully planned and structured. Even the more able person with autism will
need extra time and care to interpret the implications of any results you
give. Again, because of planning problems, your patient may not fully
grasp the implications of a given diagnosis, the need for further investigations or the likely outcome or prognosis. There is very little in the literature on breaking bad news to people with autism other than in relation to
bereavement and the death of parents, siblings or grandparents.

Doctors and others involved in disclosing any changes or abnormal findings in the patient's medical condition should discuss and prepare what they are going to say carefully beforehand. A relative or supporter should be with the person when they receive the news, unless the patient is an adult and has expressly asked for the matter to be discussed in private. Extra time will be needed to talk through the situation. In times past, bad news often wasn't shared with people who had autism because it was thought they should be protected from such news or because it was assumed that they were unlikely to understand what was being told to them.

You will need to have as much knowledge as possible about your patient's usual coping strategies and about how they are likely to respond to the news. Be clear in any distinction between what is good and bad news and if necessary break down the news into more digestible parts and take more time over its delivery. I know of one grandmother with autism who on hearing she had an ovarian cyst immediately assumed she would die of the condition. She became very distressed and agitated and took some days to calm down before she was sufficiently well enough to have the treatment options and likely diagnosis discussed with her. Staff saw her problems as largely to do with having an anxious and pessimistic personality but came to realise that she was unable to work through in her mind the implications of what was happening to her body and what relevance (in this case, ultrasound) investigations had in relation to her future well-being.

## Admission to hospital as an in-patient for surgery or medical care

### Preparing for admission

Where admission becomes necessary as a result of acute illness or accident the primary responsibility for transferring the patient will rest with staff in accident and emergency or a designated admissions unit for medicine or surgery. Some hospitals also have admission wards attached to the emergency department where patients stay for a short time before decisions about further treatment or formal admission to hospital are made. Admission for 'elective' (i.e. non-urgent) treatment, for example to an orthopaedic or other specialist department, will usually allow more time for forward planning.

Whatever the situation, staff will have to make sure that everyone involved in the patient's care is informed of the patient's particular difficulties in communicating and relating to others, and that care plans are appropriately documented with any special areas of concern. It can be helpful for the hospital if relatives, or indeed the patient, bring or carry with them a leaflet giving information on the autism spectrum and how it affects people. These are obtainable from the National Autistic Society here in the UK and presumably from other national autism organisations.

I always suggest that a copy is attached securely in a prominent place in the patient's notes so that health professionals unfamiliar with autism can immediately access an outline of the condition. Another copy should be held at the nurses' station for quick and easy reference. Admissions staff and ward clerks should also be aware of autism so that they are sensitive to the need for next of kin to check regularly on their relative's progress.

When allocating a member of the nursing staff to admit the patient formally, care should be taken to see that the nurse is aware of any potential problems, that the admissions process will best be conducted in a quiet place away from distractions and that it may be necessary to have a relative or carer on hand who knows them well to 'interpret'. If the patient lives in supported or residential accommodation, their key worker will normally accompany them to hospital. People with Asperger's syndrome or high functioning autism who live independently may not have anyone they can rely on for this; while for some the admissions process won't be a problem, for some it will. You need to take care to check their 'comfort' level with answering questions before you carry on with the normal admissions procedure.

For most people affected by autism, the procedure will have to take place in several stages. The normal expectation of answering a lot of personal questions, having weight, blood pressure, temperature and other baseline observations taken, and perhaps giving a urine sample (as is the normal expectation) may be difficult for your patient to attempt in one session. Your patient's perception of what is happening to them may be muddled and confused, and as each action requires the ability to plan and execute several different actions, none of which may be familiar or under-stood, the best approach may be to break down each part of the process into manageable small steps. I will come to this in more detail in Chapter 5 when I examine the nursing skills needed to help the patient with autism.

## Preparing for surgery

This is a particularly difficult area of concern. If the person with autism doesn't understand what is involved in surgery, where do practitioners begin to communicate what is to happen? One ground-breaking study reported in the journal *Paediatric Anaesthesia* demonstrates the great success of a management programme specifically designed to enable children with autism to be admitted for medical and surgical procedures (Van der Walt and Moran 2001). The programme was devised because of the great difficulties experienced by clinicians in trying to manage such children using normal procedures.

The authors recognised that children with autism are a neglected group with well-defined needs that have not been adequately considered in the anaesthetic literature.

They set about rectifying this by setting up a system that identified these children in advance and that alerted anaesthetic staff to the fact that the children would be attending for surgery. Management guidelines and specialist pre-admission procedures (including an Autistic Anaesthetic Questionnaire) are used to elicit specific responses regarding the nature and severity of the child's autism condition (such as severity; develop-mental level; likes/fetishes/dislikes; phobias for food, drink, activities and objects; special needs; medication; general health; and social/home circumstances). The admission process is individualised to meet the specific needs of the patient. An anaesthesia plan is drawn up and parents consulted. Decisions are made regarding special admission needs, type of pre-medication, induction of anaesthesia and post-operative strategies, and these are shared with the nurse in charge of the unit admitting the patient.

Children who are more severely affected by autism may be managed in a special quiet room adjacent to theatre. Because many of the admis-sion details are dealt with in advance the process is managed more quickly. The child is admitted only 45 minutes before surgery (thus reducing the anxiety-provoking waiting time) and is usually scheduled to be first on the operating list for the day.

Where overnight admission is planned, relatives are accommodated in a room near the child and away from the main ward, thus reducing any potential disruption to normal ward activities.

Children are given pre-operative sedatives orally in the child's favourite drink and this avoids having to use any physical restraint. Parents or carers may be given a drink at the same time (without the sedative!) to drink with the child and so encourage compliance. Routine intravenous fluids and anti-sickness prophylaxis is administered while the child is still asleep in recovery so as to minimise stress on waking. Pain relief is administered rectally also while the child is sleeping. Removal of the intravenous cannula is carried out while in recovery to ease a smooth transition to the ward. The child is discharged home as soon as possible and practical and a follow-up is carried out shortly afterwards to make sure the child is making a full recovery. (For full details of the programme and guidelines, and the anaesthetic agents involved, see Van der Walt and Moran 2001.)

The audit of the programme shows that good results are possible with a planned, co-ordinated and flexible programme and that it can both greatly reduce the need for physical restraint and improve the overall experience of admission for patients and their families. 'Parents regarded a hospital attendance as a major ordeal which our program has now effectively turned into a manageable experience for them' (Van der Walt and Moran 2001, p.405).

As staff working in general acute services begin to appreciate the difficulties experienced, it is to be hoped that more hospitals will be able to modify their practices and procedures in such a way. I haven't been able to find any similar studies relevant to adults with autism undergoing surgery despite extensive literature searches.

In the UK there is no formal 'register' of people with an autism spectrum condition, and it will be up to general practitioners or referring specialists to advise surgeons and anaesthetists about their patients' special needs. GPs should be able to access the article mentioned above quite easily, either through the internet or through their local postgraduate medical library, and may wish to discuss planned admission with the surgeon and anaesthetist beforehand. Advice may also be available from the national societies for autism. The potential to let one bad experience put off the person with autism from hospitals and doctors, or even the whole health care system, for life is a very real one, and families will be happy to involve themselves in anything that increases the chances of a positive experience.

Remember that more than one member of a family may be affected by autism (including a parent) so that when you are communicating with them they too may need extra time and attention to understand and manage the situation confronting them. They may seem overly protective or pedantic at times, or appear not to be 'taking everything in'. Make allowances for this where you can as it will help them to be more confident in helping their child and increase the chances of a successful consultation and recovery period.

## Admission to intensive care

Should the patient be admitted to intensive care, staff will need to be very alert to the needs and normal behaviours of the person with autism. The intensive care unit (ICU) of a hospital is the hub of some of the most advanced medical technology available to nursing and medical staff, and when the patient is admitted they may be bombarded with strange sensory stimuli. This has been identified in patients generally as a stress response and has been called 'ICU syndrome/delirium'.

> Signs of ICU syndrome range from disorientation to time and place, to confusion regarding the identity of their relatives, friends or even themselves. When the syndrome is severe, the patient can experience visual and auditory hallucinations, and sometimes, paranoid delusions. Patients may also experience bizarre bodily sensations: this can be seen by watching patients attempting to pluck small, invisible 'bugs' from their bodies and bedclothes. (Hardicre 2003, p.26)

Add all this to the normal sensory challenges experienced by a person with autism, and one can see that real problems could emerge for the patient, the family and the staff involved in managing their care. As Jayne

Hardicre points out, it is often the families who are most aware of what is going on in ICU, and they too require a good deal of support during this time.

> Any admission to ICU signals the fragility of human life. The daily emphasis shifts from day-to-day life, and planning the future, to survival and the corresponding desire for things to be 'as they were'. (Hardicre 2003, p.26)

Relationships between staff and families often become close, and the kind of information they receive will have an impact on their ability to cope. (Excellent advice on giving information well to people with a range of communication difficulties is covered in another article, this time by Caress 2003, which I'd recommend to nurses.) Part of managing life in ICU will be in communicating well between all parties and in being able to pre-empt any particular issues that may require careful handling because of the additional communication deficits of autism. The emotional bond between patient and nurse that often develops in ICU will also need to be thought through carefully, with nurses themselves being supported by managers in managing the many conflicting emotions that may emerge as a response to this unusual situation.

# 4 Treatment

## Obtaining consent to treatment

The problem of consent to medical procedures is a 'shadow' area from a legal point of view according to advice from the National Autistic Society's website:

> Theoretically, the autistic person, if a procedure requiring consent is recommended, and if they are conscious, should sign the consent form themselves, but in the case of most people with autism, this could not be considered to be 'informed consent'. When an emergency arises, for example if the resident [of a care home] is in acute pain, the staff need to take whatever action is in the best interests of the resident concerned in consultation with the relevant medical or dental staff. In all medical matters, staff should ensure that the parents are fully informed and consulted as appropriate.

In this case the advice is offered in relation to staff and residents of people normally resident in NAS-managed accommodation, but it would seem to make sense generally. The area becomes more complex when people with autism who live independently wish to make an autonomous decision (as is their right), but who don't appear to fully comprehend the implications of a decision or its potential outcomes.

The law here in the UK appears to assume that in personal matters parents or carers will always act in the best interests of their relative or client and that doctors will be expected to use their medical knowledge also to act in the best interests of their patient. Discretion and extreme care will need to be taken to make sure that this applies, especially where differences in statute or interpretation of the law might apply (for example, differing law in the constituent parts of the UK). Where a conflict arises between what parents want and what their child or adult relative wants, additional professional involvement and advice may be needed to clarify the position and to inform any subsequent treatment decisions (see also www.mind.org.uk for a helpful guide to the legal situation regarding consent to treatment).

## Compliance with medication and treatment decisions

Another area of huge concern is that of compliance with medication and treatment. Practitioners in both acute and primary health care services need to appreciate the myriad ways in which treatment can be compromised by an autism spectrum condition, as failure to comply is an oft-quoted reason why the health outcomes of people with autism may be perceived as less successful than for the 'neurotypical' patient.

Concepts such as 'patient-centred care', patient empowerment, patients as partners, shared decision-making and 'informed choice' all illustrate the emancipation of the patient in recent years (Grol 2001). As Grol points out, from a psychological perspective more involvement of patients is seen as leading to better health outcomes, and 'from an epidemiological viewpoint, patients are seen as rational beings who can, after being informed about the benefits and risks of treatment alternatives, decide on optimal management of their condition' (p.xvi).

Encouraging compliance with medication and treatment may be reasonably straightforward from the physician's or surgeon's perspective, given that they have been asked for their professional opinion and have offered it to the patient in good faith. This, however, fails to take account of the much wider debate in health care concerning the limitations of different 'models' of care for individual patients and the extent to which scientifically 'rational' and biologically driven approaches succeed in meeting felt needs. The 'medical model' of care has been criticised for focusing too closely on bodily processes and identified 'pathology' at the (reported) expense of other issues, any of which may impinge on the sick person's ability to recover from whatever 'illness' ails them. Once you add autism to the clinical picture, and the obvious power imbalance between the 'expert' professional and the un-knowing patient, the issue becomes rather more complicated and fraught with potential ethical issues.

When helping and caring for the person with autism, then, consideration may need to extend beyond the medical model for additional ways in which the person inside the autism label can be helped to make sense of their health problems and achieve the relevant coping strategies. It is only when this has been attempted that the chances of informed consent (or informed refusal) can begin to take place. If it becomes clear that your patient does not understand the procedure or intervention planned, it may be necessary to obtain expert advice on how best to proceed, both in terms of dealing with the communication difficulty and in terms of acknowledging the legal and moral rights of the patient to refuse treatment.

Guidelines on assessing intellectual understanding and comprehension may need to be modified to take into account the patient's particular difficulties in perception and cognition, and a clinical psychologist may need to be consulted to add to the patient's and family's own understanding of the situation and to inform good medical and health care practice. Never be tempted to take the view that the person who is having difficulty in communicating is unable to comprehend the situation just because they don't have the vocabulary necessary to comply in the normal way. They may have an alternative way of showing their approval or disapproval, and you may need to work with carers, key workers or parents as well as the patient to determine their views on a given situation. Help may also need to be obtained from a recognised advocacy service. As Teasdale (1998) has explained, there is an unspoken obligation on the part of patients to co-operate during illness that can make it difficult for individuals to speak out or argue against the type of treatment or care on offer, especially where services aren't paid for directly. Professionals organise their patients' day according to routines that suit the institution's work, restricting the amount of contact with people from the world outside hospital. Anyone who doesn't conform or accept this role runs the risk of being viewed as an 'unpopular patient' (Stockwell 1984; see also Allen 2003).

The person with autism may not appreciate that they are only one of many other patients being helped or treated and may react to physical interventions at a visceral, instinctive level. All staff involved in caring for the patient with autism will need to be aware of this and be prepared to modify their usual practice accordingly. This means not taking for granted that access to the patient's body for examination or treatment will be granted in the usual way. The patient will need extra support and explanation, and approaches will need to be as gentle and quiet as possible (for advice on this, see previous chapters).

The more able, rule-bound patients will be relatively easy to care for, provided they have understood and accepted the reasons for the actions of the health professional treating them. In the confused, uncommunicative patient, it may be harder to see immediately what can be done to reduce the tension. Parents and people who know your patient well can once again be an enormous help here, particularly in preparing for a longer stay in hospital.

## Administration of medicines

Take extreme care over the administration of medicines. Adults and children with autism may not tolerate medicines well, and alternative forms of administration may be needed. The ward pharmacist may need to liaise closely with a nominated relative, nursing staff and the prescribing doctors so that sensory sensitivities are taken into account. A preference for liquid over tablet medication may be accommodated with some substances and some may be crushable or added to food if this is more palatable and doesn't affect absorption of the medicine.

Never leave medications/drugs trolleys even momentarily unattended near the patient. Never leave tablets or liquids close by to be taken after food – always stay with the patient to ensure that the prescribed medication is taken properly and completely. Staff unfamiliar with the patient should always check the patient's identification bracelet (assuming he or she tolerates wearing one!). Never rely on the patient affirming their own identity – I know this sounds absurd, but some people with autism rely on very few words to get by. He or she may say yes or no indiscriminately if confused or disorientated, and may agree to anything if sufficiently distraught!

Some people with autism have quite severe food intolerances, or strong preferences for certain food textures, and so may be limited in what they can tolerate or what they choose to eat (see Chapter 5). This can be relevant to the administration of certain medicines or nutritional supplements and to the successful administration of surgical or pre-investigation anaesthesia.

Clearly, needles are a potential hazard, and while some people with autism can understand and accept the need for injections, you should approach giving injections with extreme care and observe your patient carefully for their response.

Rubbing furiously at the injection site or attempting to 'wash off' the substance injected has been described to me by parents. If the patient requires regular injections because of a chronic condition (such as diabetes or blood coagulation problems), it may help to approach this as a kind of ritual and to build in small, tangible rewards for its successful completion. Self-administration may be possible in the more able person with autism, but even then they may become rather obsessive about the procedure (becoming distressed if the medication is not available exactly when it is due, for example). Routines in hospital vary greatly according to demands on staff at any particular time, but this may not be appreciated by your patient who finds deviation from his or her routine potentially distressing.

Be aware that your patient may not be able to describe or explain any unwanted side-effects from their medication as other patients might. Be alert for abnormal reactions to substances and record them and get appropriate advice as soon as you suspect there may be a problem. Remember that it is not the ability to feel that is compromised by autism, but the ability to express those feelings in socially appropriate and comprehensible ways. I mention this again here because in gauging a reaction to illness and 'feeling better' in your patient, you may have to observe more carefully than usual to detect subtle nuances and changes in their clinical condition.

One very skilled autism trainer I know likens having autism to finding oneself stranded in a foreign country with no knowledge of the language, traditions or customs of the place, no map or directions, and no guidebooks to follow. You may not even recognise the country! Empathising is difficult but necessary to try to engage with the complex kinds of difficulties your patient is experiencing. I've found this analogy a useful way of thinking about things from the patient's perspective and in helping to devise strategies to help people with autism 'interpret' and 'translate' particular actions on the part of health professionals. It reminds us that many of the things we do daily as part of our taken-for-granted experience as practitioners rely greatly on passivity and mutual co-operation, neither of which can be safely assumed when caring for the patient with autism.

## Pain management

I have mentioned already that people with autism may experience unusual pain reactions. They may seem hyper- or hyposensitive to different stimuli, which has implications for any subsequent pain management strategy. This applies not only to post-operative pain and wound management but also to the management of any chronic conditions they may have or in their responses to accidents and personal injury. Self-stimulating behaviours and a tendency towards clumsiness from poor motor skills can increase the chances of accidents or opportunistic infections.

Pain is a highly complex phenomenon. It presents many 'puzzles' to nurses and other health care practitioners, because it often defies what scientists view as 'rational explanations'. As authors Fordham and Dunn (1994) have explained, some individuals fail to feel pain at all; and some pathological conditions result in the loss of ability to feel pain (such as diabetic neuropathy). Pain can be experienced without an apparent cause; can be felt in parts of the body that have been amputated (so-called 'phantom pain'); can be excruciating even where this is minimal tissue damage; can be absent following massive injuries; can be felt far away from the site of the tissue damage, sometimes all round the body or even shifting round the body. Nerve damage can result in changes of pain sensation.

In people with a condition resulting from neurological damage (as in autism) it therefore shouldn't be surprising that pain is often difficult to relate and may be experienced differently. It is often the case that when people with autism are very distressed they self-inflict pain or injury, sometimes without appearing to 'feel' the pain. Sometimes they seem actively to seek it out (head-banging for example).

Again, I could find no specific advice on pain management for people with autism in the literature, so can give little evidence-based advice on what is appropriate for a given situation. All I can do here is alert practitioners to the possibility that standard pharmacological responses to pain may be insufficient to the task of relieving pain in individuals with autism, and that a particularly careful history may be needed to work out a clinically effective treatment.

There are of course problems of reporting and interpretation to be dealt with. The usual rule that nurses are driven by 'that pain is what the patient says it is' may or may not be applicable. Difficulties in describing the site, intensity and longevity of pain is a real problem for doctors and nurses attempting to treat the patient, particularly if the person affected is unable to locate the pain using expressive hand gestures. Sometimes a general agitation is all they have to go on.

Staff working in residential care who work with a range of people affected by autism can provide useful tips and strategies here. Sometimes it is ill-fitting clothes or shoes that are the problem, or dental pain that causes the most anxiety.

Pain due to generalised infection (such as influenza) or a sore throat may present as something completely different, and it may take quite a bit of gentle verbal probing to find out where the problem lies. It can be helpful to know exactly what the person was doing before the pain came. One young man I know complained of a head pain for several days, and staff only realised the problem when they found out that he had been playing football and had been practising heading the ball. Although time had passed, the memory of the pain at the time stayed with the person (almost like a pain 'imprint') and was remembered for some time afterwards. Carers and professionals need to be alert to unusual pain responses in people (particularly children) with autism and aware of the possibility of such problems.

The normal over-the-counter pain relievers such as paracetamol seem to be well tolerated by people I know with autism, and I do know that (as with most people) injections are the least-favoured option. Given the many different types of pain experienced across chronic as well as acute conditions, there is doubtless a good doctoral study to be undertaken by an enthusiastic pharmacist in devising some basic strategies for managing pain in the person with autism.

# 5 Nursing Care Issues

## Nursing care and the patient with an autism spectrum disorder

In their exposition of what it means to be an effective nurse, Benner, Tanner and Chesla (1996) critically examine the notions of 'getting it right' and 'getting it wrong' in relation to involvement with patients and families. They explain that nurses have an elaborate discourse about the right kind, level and amount of involvement with patients and their families.

> Getting it right (being in a good relationship) is, however, typically told in terms of being in tune with the patient family needs and wishes, examining early warning signs of harm or danger, facilitating the next step in recovery, understanding and coaching, and being able in some situations just to be present in silence and tears. (Benner 1996, p.243)

As teachers and facilitators of nursing, they recognise that no nurse gets it right all of the time. In complex human relationships and practice, they know that there is no way to do well without sometimes doing poorly. Doing well, however, requires skill and moral vision – the kind that comes from 'moral dialogue and engaged confrontation within particular clinical situations' (p.243). Nursing the patient with autism well, therefore, draws on this kind of engagement with practice and with the moral endeavour to do what is best in the interests of the patient given their needs and personal aspirations.

Conceptual models of nursing that have been devised to guide nursing practice attempt to distil the essence of nursing by allowing for the nature of people; the causes of problems likely to require nursing intervention; the nature of assessment and nursing diagnosis, planning and goal-setting; the focus of intervention when implementing the care plan; the nature of evaluation; and the role of the nurse in bringing all of these aspects of nursing together (see Aggleton and Chalmers 2000). In identifying the model of nursing most appropriate to caring for a patient with autism, the nurse concerned will need to appreciate the sheer pervasiveness of the communication deficit in autism.

Psychiatrist Lorna Wing explains that studies of normal early development in babies show that there is a built-in interest in other human beings, especially, at first, in the mother or primary care-giver. 'There is also a drive to communicate in every possible way, through bodily movements and baby noises, before speech begins, and to respond to communications from others' (Wing 2001, p.4). Pretend games and imagination help to improve the child's skill in understanding other people that is so necessary for integration into social life. People with autism, however, have an inability to draw on past memories and present events to make sense of experiences, to predict what is likely to happen in the future and to make plans accordingly: '...the more complex the incoming information,' Wing advises, 'the harder it is for an individual with an autistic disorder to understand' (p.5).

Expectations of the usual nurse–patient relationship based on social interaction and co-operation and a shared opportunity to make sense of the illness experience are therefore a challenge to the person whose abilities in these areas are severely restricted. Models of care chosen will have to reflect this and emphasise the value of alternative means of communication.

The previous chapters contain the basic information required to communicate with your patient. If as a nurse you have no previous experience or knowledge of autism, you should read these, together with some of the recommended key reading that appears at the end of the book. I have included authoritative and easily digestible key reading because I know how difficult it is for busy health professionals to find enough time to undertake all the continuing professional development activities they would like and feel they need to.

Literature searches and reviews can of course be helpful, but I have found that the national autism societies provide more easily accessible information than some of the standard nursing/medical information retrieval systems, simply because they are more autism specific and user-friendly. A lot of the research into autism over the years has tended to be highly theoretical and scientific and related to educational and diagnostic rather than health care intervention per se. It is often hard to extract the nuggets of useful practical information needed to provide immediate solutions to 'here and now' problems facing practitioners in health care. The 'fog index' or complexity of language used is also quite overwhelming and befuddling at times, unless you have specific training or a background in clinical psychology and neurology.

It is not unknown for medical and other health professionals to have very high functioning autism themselves. Sometimes when they come to read the literature on autism, they begin to recognise and gain insight into some of their own problems with social and personal relationships.

For many patients with autism, effective nurse–patient communication will involve including parents, families and supporters as much as possible in trying to elicit what it is that your patient is trying to tell you. Even where language exists, it may be complex, stilted and over-formal, and apparent level of vocabulary can't always be relied upon to give an accurate indication of understanding. Together you will have to find ways of responding to your patient's unique profile and to their particular cognitive problems.

The literature on access to health care for people with learning disabilities continues to grow and to be included within government policies and programmes, but much less attention has been paid to the health care needs of people with autism, which has tended to be confined to the specialist literature in the field of autism.

It is hardly surprising then that practitioners working in general medicine and surgery don't often demonstrate the kind of knowledge and understanding necessary to support people with autism in accessing health care or undergoing treatments. This may have led to a dependence on sedation and physical restraint in helping patients with autism undergo clinical investigations and surgery, both of which can bring problems and unexpected consequences if practitioners are unfamiliar with the condition and its potential to influence clinical outcomes.

Skill and sensitivity in observing the patient will therefore be needed to see where a particular individual's vulnerabilities lie. One nursing model that I have found helpful is the 'activities of living' model devised by Roper, Logan and Tierney (1996). The five main components of the model are described as: 1. the activities of living (ALs), 2. lifespan, 3. the dependence/independence continuum, 4. factors influencing ALs and 5. individuality in living. The activities of living are:

- maintaining a safe environment
- communicating
- breathing
- eating and drinking
- eliminating (i.e. discharging bodily waste)
- personal cleansing and dressing
- controlling body temperature
- mobilising
- working and playing
- expressing sexuality
- sleeping
- dying.

According to this model, nursing interventions promote independence as far as possible and as appropriate for the patient concerned, given the nature of their health problems and any corresponding medical diagnosis and prognosis. While the doctor works with symptoms and a medical 'history' to identify the nature of a patient's problems, nurses work more generally to interpret the ways in which symptoms, beliefs and health practices can impinge on the person's ability to engage in activities of daily living, and to address any limitations amenable to nursing action.

By relating the patient's capabilities and concerns to each of these 'activities of living', it is possible to pinpoint particular vulnerabilities. Additional care also needs to be taken to identify the ways in which autism has the potential to compromise a person's ability to function effectively in any one area (expressing sexuality may be compromised by extreme sexual naivety, for example; sleeping and resting may be affected by an unidentified sleep disorder).

Spirituality and the practice of religious faith and belief is another area where people with autism may have difficulty in being able to express themselves or be able to take spiritual comfort from as a consequence of their rigidity and concrete thinking.

## Managing personal hygiene and encouraging self-care

Eating and eliminating will clearly be compromised by any diet restrictions, unusual dietary habits or food intolerances. Any associated symptoms, such as diarrhoea, constipation and vomiting, will be harder to deal with if reciprocal communication (e.g. following nursing advice or instruction) is problematic.

Difficulties in washing, bathing and maintaining personal cleanliness will require skilled nursing intervention both to enable independence as far as is practical and to ensure a safe level of hygiene and minimise the risk of auto-infection or cross-infection. People with autism may also be more susceptible than others to food poisoning and gastric infection because of poor food and hand hygiene (particularly if they live alone).

Sensory habits such as biting or scratching may cause breaks in the skin, with the potential for infection; or bruising may be evident in response to particular injury or self-stimulating behaviours. Poor or compromised nutrition may reflect itself in vitamin deficiencies and reduced immunity or vulnerability to certain related medical conditions.

Personal cleansing and dressing will require sensitive investigation and planning. What are the patient's normal routines and habits? What methods are employed to help if he or she has difficulty in this area? An occupational therapist may have been involved in teaching personal skills. Does your patient have a personal care plan they use at other times? Does he or she normally require help with washing, dressing and going to the toilet? What are the usual arrangements for cleaning of teeth, care of teeth and spectacles or any visual or hearing aids? Dental and gum hygiene may be compromised by sensory habits and by difficulties in accessing a dentist able to understand the person's sensory difficulties.

What about hair care? Some people with autism may forget or not acknowledge different aspects of their bodies. Some scratch or pull their hair, and hair loss and irritating scalp conditions can result. The person with autism who lives alone and is unable to self-care may have untreated fungal or parasitic infections.

The management of menstruation and other gynaecological matters may require special attention and help. Selective receptivity to some signals over others may mean that pain or discomfort is not expressed in ways that nursing or other health care staff would normally understand. For example, the real problem may be an ingrown toe-nail, but the patient may instead focus on a tiny pimple on their shoulder.

Lack of inhibition may pose problems in terms of privacy and observation of the usual social conventions. If the patient hasn't learned the social rules in terms of expressing sexuality, then care will be needed to see that sexual self-stimulation such as masturbation doesn't cause additional problems while in hospital.

While self-care is encouraged, domestic and house-keeping staff should be aware of the situation and know that additional cleaning and precautions may be needed as a result of the patient's difficulty in managing their personal toilet, especially if the patient has diarrhoea or constipation. They need to know that this is related to the patient's autism profile and not deliberate and a case of just being 'dirty'. Autism has been associated with abnormalities in the gut flora, and some people with autism have reported problems with eliminating and dietary intolerance (for an assessment of the literature, see Medical Research Council 2001).

Not all patients with autism will be able to tell you when they feel nauseous or that they are going to be sick. If they have asthma, epilepsy, arthritis or diabetes, they may not be able to recognise a worsening of their symptoms and know when to ask for help or how to behave. (See Chapter 4 for more about the problem of recognising and dealing with pain.) If you have taught them a procedure on one occasion, don't expect them to retain the information or to recall it for future use as this may not happen.

Problems with 'executive functioning' (see Happ 1994) impair the ability to plan or foresee the consequences of certain actions, which means that the person with autism may have to be 'taught' the same procedure many times over.

A need for sameness and preference for ritual may mean that the patient arranges their bedside locker and personal belongings in a particular way or they become engaged in performing elaborate routines. This needs to be left alone as far as possible provided it isn't harming anyone, because it may contribute a great deal to the patient's personal coping strategy – if items have to be removed or cleaned they should be put back in exactly the same place if possible.

## Maintaining patient safety

Risk assessments should be carried out along with the nursing care plan and monitored carefully in the interests of all patients and staff. Cupboards containing dangerous substances and drugs should be kept under lock and key (including cleaning fluids in hospital kitchens). Domestic staff need to keep cleaning apparatus and fluids out of harm's way. Notices on doors and safety warnings may not be noticed or may be taken literally, so care must be taken to explain the physical boundaries beyond which your patient must not go. That said, information offered may not be retained or acted upon, so don't assume that because the patient has been warned of a danger that they will necessarily heed your advice.

Note any clear risk factors in the patient's notes and care plan and make sure that they are communicated to other staff at patient report or 'handover' time.

Doctors and paramedical staff, such as physiotherapists, occupational therapists, dieticians, counsellors, phlebotomists, and other technicians, should also be kept informed of specific risks associated with your patient. Technicians who conduct heart traces (for example) should be accompanied by a member of the nursing staff (or relative) who is familiar with the patient if the patient requests it or would appear to welcome this. Be aware that your patient is unlikely to understand the principles of cross-infection and be clear and unambiguous in your instructions as to the steps patients and carers can take to help prevent this from happening.

## Managing nutrition and eating difficulties

Dietary problems are quite common in people with an autistic spectrum condition. Advice from the hospital dietician should be obtained before admission if possible so that dietary requirements can be appropriately planned for. Some people eat an extremely restricted diet, and it is thought this may partly be a sensory problem due to intolerance of strong smells or uncomfortable textures or food that tastes 'bad' in the mouth.

Some people have difficulty handling the proteins from milk products, wheat or other grain products. For this reason diets that are gluten- and casein-free have been tried with some success (Yapko 2003). Allergies and hypersensitivity reactions have also been suggested as contributing to behavioural problems in people with autism (for a guide, see Le Breton 2001).

Inflammatory bowel disease has also been studied for its links with autism (e.g. Wakefield *et al.* 1998), although a research review in the UK by the Medical Research Council (2001) found the studies to be inconclusive overall. As research in this area continues, more information and advice should become available.

From a pragmatic viewpoint I will simply list below some reported problems with nutrition, digestion and eating habits that you are likely to encounter on a hospital ward.

- *Strong preferences for certain foodstuffs over others.* This may be in response to previous food intolerance or simply to everyday likes and dislikes. I know people who live only on rice krispies and water, or who will only eat baked beans placed on the edge of the plate (if placed in the middle they will not be eaten!). This is related to the preference for ritual and routine that is often found in people with autism.

- *Particular preferences over timing of meals.* This can be difficult to accommodate with ward routines. Some people with autism can become distressed and agitated if food does not appear exactly on time. You will need to be sensitive to this possibility and see if you can come to a compromise. Some hospitals have blanket policies not allowing food to be brought from home to hospital, but it may be politic to relax these rules in consultation with the ward dietician.

- *Failure to demonstrate 'table manners' and comply with other social rules or customs.* Because the person with autism usually has a poor sense of other people's needs, they may not have learned to observe the normal customs associated with eating in company. Eating with fingers or being 'messy' with food is quite common, and those severely affected may have 'pica' (a craving to eat things that normally wouldn't be eaten). They may spit out food they find unpalatable or hide it somewhere unusual. Conversely, the more able person might have strict rules of his or her own to be observed at mealtimes (having acquired a ritualistic approach), and they may react with displeasure at any obvious disregard for 'their' rules. For example, they might need utensils to be placed in a particular position and might not be able to eat until this 'need for sameness' is satisfied. Food may be eaten slowly and deliberately or extremely quickly without chewing (hence the risk of choking), so supervision of meals is advised if this is found to be a problem.

- *Failure to maintain personal hygiene.* You may need to encourage basic personal hygiene, such as washing hands before and after meals and after going to the toilet. It is helpful if a routine can be established from the beginning of a hospital admission and warning given in advance of any intention to change the routine.

- *Forgetting to drink.* The person with autism may have poor self-care skills, so you will need to ensure that they maintain adequate hydration. They may forget to drink unless prompted and it would be a good idea to maintain a fluid-intake record even where a formal fluid-balance record is not needed for clinical reasons.

One area that can cause particular problems is when preparing for surgery or other investigation requiring that the patient be 'nil by mouth'. You will need to supervise this strictly. You may also need to explain that the 'nil by mouth' order is only for a short duration, in case the person mistakes it for a permanent change and understandably becomes concerned.

## Clinical care

The care needed to tend wounds and to maintain tissue viability and appropriate care of pressure areas need not be markedly different from that of the ordinary patient, provided care has been planned on an individual basis. Attention to communication problems and any issues already raised in previous chapters should be enough to ensure that potential problems are avoided. Dressings may need to be modified to take into account the likely mobility of the patient and their usual sensory habits and preferences. Pain will need to be carefully assessed and interventions carefully documented. Good communication between members of the nursing staff can make sure that any problems are minimised and good practice shared and repeated.

If catheterisation is required because of urinary problems or surgery, special care will be needed to see that this is carried out as gently as possible or it is likely to cause extreme distress. Similarly, any invasive procedure, such as inserting chest or wound drains or cleaning wounds and attending to pressure area care, will require very sensitive and minimal handling and close observation. Management of fever that requires clinical observations of temperature-taking, giving appropriate antipyretics and antibiotics or intravenous fluids should be carefully planned and monitored.

You may sometimes need to substitute some of the newer technologies (such as electronic methods of pulse taking and blood pressure monitoring) for more traditional manual methods if your patient is conscious and sensitive to the relatively strong pressure of the machines. Glass thermometers should never be used in the mouth as they may be resisted and chewed or bitten. Patients will normally need to be cared for by at least two nursing staff together if they are febrile and unwell, for they may be very restless and agitated and unable to understand what is being done to help them.

The standard use of extractor and cooling fans and sponging down to help a patient with fever may have to be dealt with differently if the patient is distressed or anxious.

Measurement of fluid balance and taking of urine or stool samples or special tests will need to be meticulously explained and careful note taken of any accidents or associated problems.

Topical skin treatments used need to be assessed for the possibility of accidental ingestion (one lady I know was used to literally 'licking her wounds'), and supervision of administration needs to be continued until treatment has finished. A personal planner can be devised for patients taking medication home with them, but care should be taken to make sure that administration is still supervised, both in the number and timing of applications. Hygiene measures should also be put in place, as some people with autism may not bathe or clean themselves regularly in the normal way, and so delay healing. I know of one boy who only washes his front (not being aware of the rest of his body). Rates of healing may vary due to other factors (particularly self-injury).

## Sleep disorders and 'night-time wandering'

Nursing staff should be aware that many people with autism have difficulty sleeping.

Staff working on nights should be prepared for this in caring for the patient with autism. Such children and adults seem to have no difficulty managing on very little sleep. It is often the people living with or caring for them that suffer from true sleep 'deprivation'. Clearly there is the potential for lack of sleep to interfere with physical and mental health, so that where normal strategies for encouraging sleep don't work, specialist advice is sought from one of the support organisations. Many parents and partners don't have regular access to respite facilities, and it is only when the person is admitted to hospital that sleep problems are properly recognised and investigated.

Severely affected people may not distinguish night from day and take to wandering at night. The implications for general patient safety should be taken into account here, as patients could easily become disorientated and disturb other patients on the ward. Night sedation may have the effect of disorientating the patient further, leading to additional confusion and distress, so expert advice (taking into account his or her normal sleep routines) should be obtained as to the best way forward. Sometimes unwillingness to sleep will be due to anxiety or a specific worry or sensory intrusion (a light left on or off, the sound of oxygen bubbles or bleeping of a drip monitor) that can be identified and addressed.

Pain may also complicate the situation. Sutures or bandages may be very uncomfortable and be felt as very heavy pressure, which the person then attempts to dislodge. Careful observation should elicit any external factors. Sometimes your patient will be hungry or thirsty but unable to vocalise their needs. If it is safe to do so, let him or her show you or lead you to what they want, although this may be more difficult if the environment is strange to them or they have different tubes and machines attached to them. Access to any special toys or interests (including special interest magazines) may enable them to rest quietly. Night-time wandering and alertness is not at all unusual, so be sure to make enquiries prior to admission if possible so that you can plan for this and place the patient in the most suitable room and close to nursing supervision.

## Social aspects of being a hospital patient

In terms of managing the 'self' and the role of patient in hospital, do remember that sensitivity to normal social conventions is unlikely to occur to your patient with autism unless he or she is very able and has learned to recognise social cues through teaching or trial and error. The normal respect for privacy, not listening or joining in on private conversations or consultations, and being appropriately respectful if a fellow patient has had a bad experience or there has been a death on the ward will provide substantial challenges to their social skills.

For people with high functioning autism, talking at length about a subject of their choosing and with little obvious regard for the people listening is a normal event. They may need to receive some clear reminders about what is appropriate to their situation and to be asked to 'save up' what they want to say or do until a more appropriate time.

As a caveat to this it is worth noting, however, that a person's special interest may be a sign of increasing anxiety, and any sudden intense return to it may signal that the patient is attempting to find a temporary refuge away from whatever may be worrying them or causing them pain.

If this appears to be the case, try to help the person explain or relax in whatever ways seem appropriate to the situation. When my son was young, he used to immerse himself in Star Trek videos, and we soon came to recognise this as a kind of 'tuning out' into a private safe space where he could psychologically cut himself off from whatever was making him anxious. Any withdrawal into a special interest should be assessed and monitored for any signs that a perceived or actual problem requires attention.

Staying in hospital, away from familiar people and things, is hard for most people to deal with. One of the ways in which patients cope is by taking a polite interest in their fellow patients and by chatting to them or helping them out informally (if they are well enough) during a hospital stay. But be constantly aware that one of the most stressful things you can do to a person with autism is expect them to socialise. In the normal hospital situation patients are often expected to chat with their neighbour in the next bed. In some cases patients become very familiar and form friendships that last beyond the period of hospitalisation. The demands on one's social skills as a fellow patient can be great, however, especially in wards that have four-bedded bays and where a degree of intimacy can't be avoided.

People with Asperger's syndrome can be very taxing if they fail to recognise normal social boundaries in terms of physical space (standing or sitting too close, talking too loudly or too quickly, staring or failing to maintain appropriate eye contact, constantly interrupting or butting in on private conversations, offering frank opinions and assessments of other people's situations and personal appearances, which may not be welcomed!). When patients are sick and in need of rest, they may not be able to summon the social skills necessary to 'manage' your patient with autism, especially at night and when nursing staff are not immediately on hand to help. It isn't really fair to expect them to.

From my own experience as a hospital patient I have often found the task of reassuring other patients and being a confidante to them a challenge to my own good manners – not because I dislike people or I don't have the necessary social skills, but because my emotional and physical reserves of energy were, owing to illness, simply not up to the job.

Hospitals are notoriously noisy and difficult places to rest in and nursing staff are not always aware of the tensions this can cause. Sensitivity to the situation and a careful assessment of coping skills are therefore necessary to avoid clashes or bad feeling. If a single room is available, think about what I have written previously and try to assess the best option for your patient, bearing in mind the emotional energies and personalities involved. If the patient is being cared for in a single room, constant supervision may be necessary, or he or she may decide it is time to go home or venture elsewhere, regardless of their current medical condition or any medical equipment that may be attached to their person. They are unlikely to leave you a note of where they have gone, so don't be tempted to skimp on supervision!

## The dying patient and autism

I have not been able to find any detailed autism-specific information or literature that addresses this issue directly in the time that I have been researching material for this book. Clearly it would be an area for further research and exploration, particularly as it has been suggested that there are a fair number of people with autism who spend a lot of time thinking about death and death-related themes (Gillberg 2002). Palliative care services tend to be most associated with cancer, but the experiences of patients dying from other conditions is beginning to be acknowledged and services modified.

As more personal accounts are published, understanding may increase; and individuals and families affected by bereavement, or who have been advised they have a terminal illness, should ask their family doctors for support and advice.

## Discharge planning and aftercare

Discharge and aftercare should be planned in the normal way, although it may be necessary to have home assessments carried out if the person being discharged has new medical needs that will require adaptation. Occupational therapy expertise is likely to be very useful (particularly if there is expertise in sensory impairments).

Newly diagnosed medical conditions that require monitoring and follow-up should be communicated to the appropriate professionals in the community health care team.

Community and practice nurses now often run specialist clinics for a range of conditions (coronary heart disease, asthma, diabetes being the first examples that spring to mind), and an appropriate referral could certainly improve the chances of the person's aftercare being adequately supervised. Advice from community psychiatric and learning disability staff or child and adolescent health care teams may be available if appropriate (although specific knowledge about autism may still be rather patchy and inconsistent).

I could find very little in the literature regarding the management of chronic medical conditions in community practice for people with autism (for a very helpful account on supporting adults with autism and specific health needs, see Morgan 1996). The management of chronic medical conditions has developed a great deal in recent years in partnership with patients, and it would be very valuable to see further exploration of strategies to help people with autism manage such conditions as asthma, diabetes, chronic fatigue syndrome, arthritis, cancer, and all the other debilitating conditions encountered in everyday practice (another book, alas!).

# 6 Social Support

## Support for families and carers

Carers and families need support not only during a period of hospitalisation for their relative with autism, but also in day-to-day living. Staff working in community or residential settings recognise that working with people with autism can be draining, physically and emotionally, but also very rewarding. They also know, however, that (residential care workers excepted) they can go home at the end of their shift or working hours and recoup energy given up at work.

Most of the families I know don't have regular access to respite facilities, so the experience is continuous, and can become lifelong if their dependent child grows up to become a dependent adult with little access to the few appropriate leisure facilities and employment.

When the child is young, respite may only be for a few hours a day (less if parents choose and are supported to educate their child at home). Adolescence is a particularly trying time for most young people as they test out the normal boundaries between childhood and adulthood and as they come to rely on peers and friends as confidants and companions.

Where a young person has not been able to secure friendships (or even any friendship) or a coherent social network, reliance on the family becomes even greater. This can cause internal strains as the family dynamic tries to adjust to new demands.

As Richard Howlin explains, by adolescence the person with Asperger's syndrome is likely to have experienced years of social confusion and negative self-attributions, and have become highly sensitive or indifferent to peer relationships. Efforts to achieve a generalised sense of personal mastery and self-confidence are also likely to be significantly handicapped (Howlin 2003). Teenager Luke Jackson gives his personal account of AS in adolescence and shares his philosophy that to be different is 'cool', encouraging us to remember that every one of us is amazing in our own way (Jackson 2002). Not everyone I have met with autism has been able to show this level of personal acceptance of autism, however, and some use up a lot of valuable energy in 'fighting off' what usually turns out to be an inevitable return to former problems.

Staff working in health care who are familiar with the feelings of anger and denial that accompany 'bad news' should also be able to recognise some of the emotional difficulties people encounter when a person or family is affected by autism. How the family copes may depend on how the initial diagnosis was managed; on access to appropriate understanding and services; on the practical problems associated with caring for their loved one; on the kind of relationship they have with their affected relative; and on all the ordinary tensions that can affect family life.

As one young man with autism wrote eloquently on his personal web page, 'autism breaks families' hearts'. Undeniably, some families and relationships don't survive the pressures involved, and it is quite common for people with autism to live in a single-parent household with all the worries and difficulties this can bring, both emotionally and financially. Social life can become very restricted for non-affected members of the family, particularly if problems are not understood by neighbours, friends and extended family. Social skills can become blunted or 'rusty', and a disinclination to become involved in activities outside the family unit can be an easy habit to fall into. Opportunities for leisure and paid employment may be adversely affected by carer obligations. The health needs of carers may also be overlooked as the national organisations for carers are well aware.

The experience of caring for a person with autism can be lonely if the person being cared for becomes absorbed in their personal routines and interests to the exclusion of other things. It can be very 'wearing' to listen to someone's incessant monologues if you have no shared interest and little attention is paid to your own needs in turn.

Even where people have had successful relationships, extra work and understanding is needed to maintain the relationship (see an account of a successful 'Asperger marriage' in Slater-Walker and Slater-Walker 2002).

All of these factors should be taken into account when considering the needs and demands on carers, and support should be offered wherever possible. Social workers and adult support services are gradually becoming more aware of the problems associated with autism, and services are beginning to develop as a result. Again, geography and local priorities and budgets often constrain the support offered.

Informal support and self-help groups may fill the gap in some areas (and are to be recommended), although it is important not to place too much responsibility on support groups since they can easily find themselves becoming the only recognised service if formal support services are not well developed in relation to autism in their locality. The voluntary organisations do a great deal of work in this area and are probably the biggest single source of reliable information and support for people affected by autism, along with specialist publishers.

Family doctors supporting families affected by autism should recognise the different ways people cope with a diagnosis of autism. Some will grieve openly, while others will keep their worries and strains private. Mike Stanton's excellent account of learning to live with high functioning autism addresses the issue of coping strategies, and examines both the 'worrier' and the 'warrior' approaches to managing the situation (Stanton 2000). Worriers and warriors have different priorities. The first will be consumed with guilt, while the latter will be determined to get the best for their child, come what may. (I had to smile when I recognised myself in this highly insightful and empathic retelling of his own experiences.) While not wanting to suggest that parents will fall completely into either category, GPs will recognise both kinds of coping strategy – parents in denial, parents on the warpath, parents alarmed and confused and afraid for the future.

I know that some parents' initial reaction is to glean as much information as possible about autism (aided by the internet). As a branch worker for the National Autistic Society, I can often sense the rage, anger and grief of parents whose relative has been recently diagnosed. I recognise it as a natural reaction to news that has implications for a lifetime. Even some time after diagnosis, and especially as new developmental transitions are approached (e.g. going to school, puberty, leaving school or going to college, the first child leaving the family home), sadness and 'chronic sorrow' can re-emerge and the loss be newly felt as unanticipated limitations are recognised and earlier aspirations have to be rethought.

Families whose affected relative lives in supported or residential accommodation speak movingly about the feelings and conflicts they experience at different stages in transition, and particularly where there is doubt about how their relative is going to be supported after close relatives have died or when a remaining family member does not wish to take responsibility.

Admission to hospital may be a time when these worries are again brought to the fore, or existing coping and management strategies called into question. Staff in hospitals can help by listening carefully to any worries or concerns and by liaising with community support services (both statutory and voluntary) to see how best to make any proposed transition to new arrangements following hospital discharge.

If parents or carers are elderly and have needs of their own, it may gradually become obvious that existing arrangements cannot continue. Advice on benefits and formal support for daily living may be needed for the first time if the family have not had access to appropriate information and support before.

### Carers with autism

I have never seen it acknowledged anywhere that people with autism can also be carers. People with undiagnosed autism living in close-knit family units, who have lived reclusive lives and may never have come to professionals' attention, must sometimes have taken on the role of informal carers (presumably with functional limitations), and some will have developed caring abilities beyond those that might be imagined by those with a detailed knowledge of autism. Health care staff need to be alert to this potential issue, and to recognise situations that may result in people with autism becoming carers by an unexpected change in personal circumstances. No one can say, reliably, how many people with autism will find themselves in this position, nor can they say with any authority that this would be undesirable. With proper support, carers with autism may be very successful, though within the limits imposed by their communication difficulties and the severity of their autism spectrum condition.

My own son has become a 'young carer' in recent years after I was diagnosed with multiple sclerosis, and although this places no great strains on us at the present time, it may well become more of an issue in the future should my health deteriorate or should his father no longer be around to support the family as a whole.

## Bereavement and autism

Advice on autism and bereavement can be accessed from the UK National Autistic Society website, where moving accounts can be found of the different ways people with autism reflect on issues such as serious illness and bereavement.

In the past, when institutional or custodial care of more severely affected people with autism was the norm, it was sometimes thought best not to inform people of the death of relatives. We can only imagine (now that we understand more about these issues) the pain and distress that was sometimes caused to individuals because of this. Who can say whether or not for some this was the right decision? It was often made from the best of motives.

Responses to serious illness and death can depend a great deal on an individual's faith and cultural practices. Care and sensitivity will be needed by those disclosing bad news to see that the individual is properly supported and understands what is expected of them.

## Community education

Last, but not least, I would like to stress the need for continuing awareness-raising regarding autism across the community and in the helping professions. I can add dentists, social workers, community pharmacists, optometrists, citizens' advice bureaus, ambulance personnel, midwives and paramedics, first-aiders, police and legal advice agencies, firefighters, and the community as a whole as benefiting from detailed information about the ways in which autism needs to be better understood. Important publications are already beginning to address these areas (e.g. Davis and Schunick 2002; Debbaudt 2002).

# Afterword

In this book I have tried to tackle some major issues, all of which deserve much greater attention than I have been able to give in one small volume. My hope is that at least it will encourage the asking of relevant questions. Lorna Wing has done a very great deal to bring our attention to the challenges that autism spectrum conditions bring to the world. She writes:

> Those of us who live and/or work with children and adults with autistic disorders have to try to enter their world, since they cannot find their way into ours. We need to learn to comprehend and empathize with autistic experiences in order to find ways to help each individual cope with a system of social rules that is alien to them. (Wing 1996, p.225)

My fervent hope is that everyone working in health care will take some time to improve their knowledge of autism, so that never again will a parent have to apologise for what is normal and usual for their relative. As Luke Jackson says, to be different is 'cool'. As a parent and as an educator, I certainly brook no argument with that!

# APPENDIX I 'Fast Facts' about the autism spectrum

Autism and the related conditions high functioning autism and Asperger's syndrome affect (very roughly) about 1 per cent of the population.

Autism is a lifelong developmental disorder affecting social and communication skills.

The degree to which people are affected varies widely. Those with 'classic' or 'Kanner's autism' tend to be socially very withdrawn with poor language skills, while those with high functioning autism or Asperger's syndrome may use very complicated language but still have the same innate difficulty in relating to people and understanding the needs and intentions of others.

Autism is due to abnormalities of brain function, but so far no clear single cause has been identified.

More than one member of a family can be affected.

Children with autism become adults with autism.

There is currently no cure for the condition, although people can be greatly helped by understanding, support and access to advice from speech and language therapists, occupational therapists, teachers and social workers who are trained in the specific problems experienced by those with the condition.

Many people with autism are very sensitive to touch or sound, so access to special sensory rooms or play areas can be very comforting.

Conversely, they may seem insensitive to pain stimuli that other people would find distressing. Such sensory integration problems have huge implications for health care and should be noted by practising health professionals.

Diagnosis is made by recognising characteristic patterns of behaviour present from early in life (Wing 1996).

Diagnostic criteria for autism spectrum conditions have broadened in recent years in response to extensive research in the autism field. Specialist opinions vary as to the range of conditions included on the autism spectrum but always include those mentioned above.

There are now many more people trained to recognise and diagnose autism, hence an apparent increase in the prevalence. As awareness increases, more adults are receiving a diagnosis of Asperger's syndrome.

Diagnostic practices vary depending on local services and who has received appropriate training. Psychiatric, paediatric and multi-professional assessment is usually undertaken before a confident diagnosis can be made.

Many children and young people with autism are now educated in mainstream schools and colleges, and intellectually able people with autism attend university with variable levels of support. Access to specialist schooling for children with autism depends on geography and availability of resources.

Very few people with moderate to severe autism currently go on to full-time work or enjoy long-term relationships or marriage, although this may change with greater social awareness and understanding.

*For more detailed answers to the most frequently asked questions from health care staff I have provided a list of accessible key reading (Appendix 2).*

# Key reading and resources

The range of books and other resources available on autism and Asperger's syndrome has increased enormously over the past five years and is improving all the time. Included below is a short list that I and colleagues and friends have found helpful. There are cultural differences in the way autism is dealt with in the literature, depending on the way people with autism are stereotyped and the causes people attribute to the condition. Some attitudes have been acquired historically, while media coverage of other possible contributing factors can also affect the therapeutic approaches taken to improve communication skills and quality of life.

My personal journey has led me to believe that autism is largely genetically acquired, together with exposure to some significant clinical hazards both before and after birth. The list below probably reflects this bias but also includes references to works that explore a range of issues in the autism field.

## Books

Aarons, M. and Gittens, T. (1999) *The Handbook of Autism: A Guide for Parents and Professionals*. London: Routledge.

Attwood, T. (1993) *Why Does Chris Do That?* London: National Autistic Society.

Attwood, T. (1998) *Asperger's Syndrome: A Guide for Parents and Professionals*. London: Jessica Kingsley Publishers.

Bauman, M.L. and Kemper, T.L. (eds) (1997) *The Neurobiology of Autism*. Baltimore, MD: Johns Hopkins University Press.

Clements, J. and Zarkowska, E. (2000) *Behavioural Concerns and Autistic Spectrum Disorders*. London: Jessica Kingsley Publishers.

Frith, U. (1991) *Autism and Asperger Syndrome.* Cambridge: Cambridge University Press.

Frith, U. (2003) *Autism: Explaining the Enigma.* Oxford: Blackwell.

Gillberg, C. (2002) *A Guide to Asperger Syndrome* Cambridge: Cambridge University Press.

Gray, C. (1995) 'Teaching children with autism to "read" social situations.' In K.A. Quill (ed) *Teaching Children with Autism: Strategies to Enhance Communication and Socialization.* New York: Delmar.

Gray, C. and Leigh White, A. (2002) *My Social Stories Book.* London: Jessica Kingsley Publishers.

Howlin, P. (1997) *Autism: Preparing for Adulthood.* London: Routledge.

Howlin, P. (1998) *Children with Autism and Asperger Syndrome.* Chichester: Wiley.

Jackson, L. (2002) *Freaks, Geeks and Asperger Syndrome: A User Guide to Adolescence.* London: Jessica Kingsley Publishers.

Peeters, T. and Gillberg, C. (1999) *Autism: Medical and Educational Aspects.* London: Whurr.

Rankin, K. (2000) *Growing Up Severely Autistic.* London: Jessica Kingsley Publishers.

Whitaker, P., Joy, H., Harley, J. and Edwards, D. (2001) *Challenging Behaviour and Autism – Making Sense, Making Progress.* London: National Autistic Society.

Wing, L. (2001) *The Autistic Spectrum: A Parents' Guide to Understanding and Helping Your Child.* Berkeley, CA: Ulysses Press.

Wing, L. (2003) *The Autistic Spectrum: A Guide for Parents and Professionals.* London: Constable & Robinson.

Yapko, D. (2003) *Understanding Autism Spectrum Disorders: Frequently Asked Questions.* London: Jessica Kingsley Publishers.

## Factsheets

A range of very useful factsheets is available online from the UK National Autistic Society (www.nas.org.uk). Those written for health professionals include:

'Diagnostic options: A guide for health professionals'

'Autism and genetics: A briefing paper'

'Mental health and Asperger syndrome'

'Autistic spectrum disorders: An introduction for general practitioners'

The website also has access to research in progress and an online enquiry service.

For the address and contact details of the NAS Publications Department either see the website given above or contact the NAS Information Centre below.

The NAS Information Centre, which runs a current awareness service and holds a database of autism publications, can be called on 020 7903 3599. The NAS Helpline number for parents and general enquiries is 0870 600 8585.

Health professionals may like to begin by reading the Medical Research Council's *Review of Autism Research: Epidemiology and Causes* (2001), which discusses many of the contentious issues and debates. For a discussion on issues regarding diagnosis, see Baird, Cass and Slonims (2003) referenced below.

## Journals

Professional journals include:

*Journal of Autism and Developmental Disorders* (published by Kluwer Academic/Plenum Publishers: Kluwer Academic Publishers, 101 Philip Drive, Assinipi Park, Norwell, MA 02061, USA)

*Good Autism Practice* (published by the British Institute of Learning Disabilities, Campion House, Green Street, Kidderminster, Worcestershire DY10 1JL)

*Autism: The International Journal of Research and Practice* (a quarterly published jointly with the UK National Autistic Society by Sage Publications, 6 Bonhill Street, London EC2A 4PU; or in North America from Sage Publications Inc., PO Box 5096, Thousand Oaks, CA 91359, USA)

## Websites

The NAS website (www.nas.org.uk) has contact information on autism societies across the world as well as giving information on local UK branches and specialist educational establishments.

For an extensive and up-to-date range of websites and helpful organisations see Yapko (2003) above. Diane Yapko's book would be invaluable on a health professional's bookshelf – it provides authoritative information and very accessible answers to the questions parents ask in response to continuing media attention and concerns about the apparent rise in diagnosis of autism and related disorders.

The website of Jessica Kingsley Publishers is also very useful for keeping up with the latest reading in the field (www.jkp.com).

# References

Aarons, M. and Gittens, T. (1999) *The Handbook of Autism: A Guide for Parents and Professionals*. London: Routledge.

Aggleton, P. and Chalmers, H. (2000) *Nursing Models and Nursing Practice*. Basingstoke: Palgrave.

Allen, D. (2003) 'Popularity stakes.' *Nursing Standard 17*, 42, 14–15.

Attwood, T. (1998) *Asperger's Syndrome: A Guide for Parents and Professionals*. London: Jessica Kingsley Publishers.

Baird, G., Cass, H. and Slonims, V. (2003) 'Diagnosis of autism – a clinical review.' *British Medical Journal 237*, August 30, 488–493. Also available from www.bmj.com

Baron-Cohen, S. (1997) *Mindblindness: An Essay on Autism and Theory of Mind*. Cambridge, MA: MIT Press.

Baron-Cohen, S. and Bolton, P. (1993) *Autism: The Facts*. Oxford: Oxford University Press.

Benner, P.A., Tanner, C.A. and Chesla, C.A. (1996) *Expertise in Nursing Practice: Caring, Clinical Judgment and Ethics*. New York: Springer.

Bingham, M. (2003) *Autism and the Human Gut Microflora*. Reading: University of Reading Food Microbial Sciences Unit.

Bolick, T. (2001) *Asperger Syndrome and Adolescence: Helping Pre-Teens and Teens Get Ready for the Real World*. Gloucester, MA: Four Winds Press.

Bornat, J. (1999) *Working with Life Experience. Block 4, Course Unit for K100 Understanding Health and Social Care*. Milton Keynes: School of Health and Social Welfare, Open University.

Brogan, C. (2001) *The Pathway to Care for Children with Autistic Spectrum Disorders*. Glasgow: NHS Greater Glasgow/National Autistic Society.

Clarke, D.J. (1996) 'Psychiatric and behavioural problems and pharmacological treatments.' In H. Morgan (ed) *Adults with Autism: A Guide to Theory and Practice*. Cambridge: Cambridge University Press.

Davis, B. and Schunick, W.G. (2002) *Dangerous Encounters – Avoiding Perilous Situations with Autism: A Streetwise Guide for all Emergency Responders, Retailers and Parents*. London: Jessica Kingsley Publishers.

Debbaudt, D. (2002) *Autism, Advocates, and Law Enforcement Professionals: Recognizing and Reducing Risk Situations for People with Autism Spectrum Disorders*. London: Jessica Kingsley Publishers.

Department of Health (2003a) *Draft Guidance on the Use of Physical Interventions for Staff Working with Children and Adults with Learning Disability and/or Autism*. www.doh.gov.uk/learningdisabilities/dgapp1.htm

Department of Health (2003b) *What to Do If You're Worried a Child is Being Abused*. Children's Services Guidance. www.doh.gov.uk/safeguardingchildren/safeguardingchildren.pdf

Donaldson, L. (2000) 'Clinical Governance: A Quality Concept.' In T. Van Zwanenberg and J. Harrison (eds) *Clinical Governance in Primary Care*. Abingdon: Radcliffe Medical Press Ltd.

Donellan, A. and Leary, M. (1995) *Movement Differences and Diversity in Autism and Mental Retardation*. Newmarket, Ontario: DRI Press.

Fordham, M. and Dunn, V. (1994) *Alongside the Person in Pain: Holistic Care and Nursing Practice*. London: Bailliere Tindall.

Gillberg, C. (2002) *A Guide to Asperger Syndrome*. Cambridge: Cambridge University Press.

Gray, S., Ruble, L. and Dalrymple, N. (2000) *Autism and Sexuality: A Guide for Instruction*. Bloomington, IN: Autism Society of Indiana.

Grol, R. (2001) 'Foreword'. In A. Edwards and G. Elwyn (eds) *Evidence-Based Patient Choice – Inevitable or Impossible?* Oxford: Oxford University Press.

Happe, F. (1994) *Autism: An Introduction to Psychological Theory*. London: UCL Press.

Hardicre, J. (2003) 'Meeting the needs of families of patients in intensive care units.' *Nursing Times 99*, 27, 26–27.

Henault, I. (2003) 'The sexuality of adolescents with Asperger syndrome.' In L. Holliday Willey (ed) *Asperger Syndrome in Adolescence: Living with the Ups, the Downs and the Things in Between*. London: Jessica Kingsley Publishers.

Holliday Willey, L. (1999) *Pretending to be Normal: Living with Asperger's Syndrome*. London: Jessica Kingsley Publishers.

Howlin, P. (1998) *Children with Autism and Asperger Syndrome: A Guide for Practitioners and Carers*. Chichester: Wiley.

Howlin, R. (2003) 'Asperger syndrome in the adolescent years.' In L. Holliday Willey (ed) *Asperger Syndrome in Adolescence: Living with the Ups, the Downs and Things in Between.* London: Jessica Kingsley Publishers.

Jackson, L. (2002) *Freaks, Geeks and Asperger Syndrome: A User Guide to Adolescence.* London: Jessica Kingsley Publishers.

Jarrold, C. and Routh, D.A. (1998) 'Is there really a link between engineering and autism? A reply to Baron-Cohen *et al.' International Journal of Research and Practice 2,* 3, 281-289.

Jones, G., Jordan, R. and Morgan, H. (2001) *All About Autistic Spectrum Disorders: A Booklet for Parents and Carers.* London: Mental Health Foundation.

Jordan, R. (1999) *Autistic Spectrum Disorders: An Introductory Handbook for Practitioners.* London: David Fulton.

Jordan, R. (2001) *Autism with Severe Learning Difficulties: A Guide for Parents and Professionals.* London: Souvenir Press.

Le Breton, M. (2001) *Diet Intervention and Autism: Implementing the Gluten Free and Casein Free Diet for Autistic Children and Adults.* London: Jessica Kingsley Publishers.

Medical Research Council (2001) *Review of Autism Research: Epidemiology and Causes.* London: Medical Research Council.

Mental Health Foundation (1994) *Legal Issues Arising from the Care, Control and Safety of Children with Learning Disabilities who also Present Severe Challenging Behaviour.* London: Mental Health Foundation.

Morgan, H. (1996) *Adults with Autism: A Guide to Theory and Practice.* Cambridge: Cambridge University Press.

Nally, B. and Bliss, V.E. (2000) *Recognising and Coping with Stress. Booklet 5, Focus on the Family Series.* London: National Autistic Society.

National Autistic Society (1999) *Factsheet: Autistic Spectrum Disorders – An Introduction for GPs.* London: National Autistic Society.

Novack, D.H. (1999) 'Foreword.' In F.W. Platt and G.H. Gordon, *Field Guide to the Difficult Patient Interview.* Philadelphia: Lippincott, Williams and Wilkins.

Radley, A. (1994) *Making Sense of Illness: The Social Psychology of Health and Disease.* London: Sage.

Roper, N., Logan, W.W. and Tierney, A.J. (1996) *The Elements of Nursing: A Model for Nursing Based on a Model of Living (4th edn).* Edinburgh: Churchill Livingstone.

Schneider, E. (1999) *Discovering My Autism: Apologia Pro Vita Sua (with Apologies to Cardinal Newman).* London: Jessica Kingsley Publishers.

Schopler, E. (1995) *Parent Survival Manual: A Guide to Crisis Resolution in Autism and Related Developmental Disorders.* New York and London: Plenum Press.

Slater-Walker, G. and Slater-Walker, C. (2002) *An Asperger Marriage.* London: Jessica Kingsley Publishers.

Smith Myles, B., Tapscott Cook, K., Miller, N.E., Rinner, L. and Robbins, L.A. (2000) *Asperger Syndrome and Sensory Issues: Practical Solutions for Making Sense of the World.* Shawnee Mission, KS: Autism Asperger Publishing.

Soltysiak, B. and O'Shea, P. (2003) 'A communication protocol to help patients with sensory impairment.' *Professional Nurse 18,* 10, 557–560.

Stanton, M. (2000) *Learning to Live with High Functioning Autism: A Parent's Guide for Professionals.* London: Jessica Kingsley Publishers.

Stockwell, F. (1984) *The Unpopular Patient.* London: Croom Helm.

Teasdale, K. (1998) *Advocacy in Health Care.* Oxford: Blackwell Science.

Tingle, J.H. (1995) 'The legal accountability of the nurse.' In R. Watson (ed) *Accountability in Nursing Practice.* London: Chapman & Hall.

Van der Walt, J.H. and Moran, C. (2001) 'An audit of perioperative management of autistic children.' *Paediatric Anaesthesia 11,* 401–408.

Wainscott, G. and Corbett, J. (1996) 'Health care of adults with autism.' In H. Morgan (ed) *Adults with Autism: A Guide to Theory and Practice.* Cambridge: Cambridge University Press.

Wakefield, A.J., Murch, S.H., Anthony, A., Linnell, J., Casoon, D.M., Malik, M., Berelowitz, M., Dhillan, A.P., Thomson, M.A., Harvey, P., Valentine, A., Davies, S.E. and Walker-Smith, J.A. (1998) 'Ileal-lymphoid-nodular hyperplasia, non-specific colitis, and pervasive developmental disorder in children.' *The Lancet 351,* 637–641.

Whitaker, P. (2001) *Challenging Behaviour and Autism – Making Sense, Making Progress: A Guide to Preventing and Managing Challenging Behaviour for Parents and Teachers.* London: National Autistic Society.

Wing, L. (1996) *The Autistic Spectrum: A Guide for Parents and Professionals.* London: Constable & Robinson.

Wing, L. (2001) *The Autistic Spectrum: A Parents' Guide to Understanding and Helping Your Child.* Berkeley, CA: Ulysses Press.

Wing, L. and Shah, A. (2000) 'Catatonia in autistic spectrum disorders.' *British Journal of Psychiatry 176,* 357–362.

Yapko, D. (2003) *Understanding Autism Spectrum Disorders: Frequently Asked Questions.* London: Jessica Kingsley Publishers.

# Subject Index

# Author Index